W0050815

# X-RAY FLUORESCENT SCANNING OF THE THYROID

DEVELOPMENTS IN NUCLEAR MEDICINE

Series editor Peter H. Cox

*Other titles in this series*

Cox, P.H. (ed.): Cholescintigraphy. 1981. ISBN 90-247-2524-0
Cox, P.H. (ed.): Progress in Radiopharmacology 3. Selected Topics. 1982.
ISBN 90-247-2768-5

# X-ray fluorescent scanning of the thyroid

*edited by*

**M.H. JONCKHEER MD, PhD**
**F. DECONINCK PhD**

*Department of Radioisotopes*
*Academic Hospital*
*Vrije Universiteit*
*Brussel*

1983 **MARTINUS NIJHOFF PUBLISHERS**
a member of the KLUWER ACADEMIC PUBLISHERS GROUP
BOSTON / THE HAGUE / DORDRECHT / LANCASTER

**Distributors**

*for the United States and Canada*: Kluwer Boston, Inc., 190 Old Derby Street, Hingham, MA 02043, USA
*for all other countries*: Kluwer Academic Publishers Group, Distribution Center, P.O.Box 322, 3300 AH Dordrecht, The Netherlands

**Library of Congress Cataloging in Publication Data**      CIP

Main entry under title:

X-ray fluorescent scanning of the thyroid.

    (Developments in nuclear medicine ; v. 3)
    Papers presented at Post-Congress Meeting on X-ray
fluorescence and the Thyroid, Brussels, Sept. 4, 1982.
    Includes indexes.
    1. Thyroid gland--Congresses. 2. Iodine--Analysis--
Congresses. 3. X-ray spectroscopy--Congresses.
4. Fluorescence spectroscopy--Congresses. I. Jonckheer,
M. H. III. Post-Congress Meeting on X-ray Fluroes-
cence and the Thyroid (1982 : Brussels, Belgium)
IV. Series. [DNLM: 1. Thyroid gland--Radiography--
Congresses. 2. Fluorescence--Congresses. W1 DE998KF
v. 3 / WK 200 X75 1982]
QP188.T54X18 1983      612'.44      83-2323
ISBN 0-89838-561-X

ISBN-13: 978-94-009-6707-6          e-ISBN-13: 978-94-009-6705-2
DOI: 10.1007/978-94-009-6705-2

**Copyright**

© 1983 by Martinus Nijhoff Publishers, Boston.
Softcover reprint of the hardcover 1st edition 1983

All rights reserved. No part of this publication may be reproduced, stored in a retrieval system, or transmitted in any form or by any means, mechanical, photocopying, recording, or otherwise, without the prior written permission of the publishers,
Martinus Nijhoff Publishers, 190 Old Derby Street, Hingham, MA 02043, USA.

# CONTENTS

FOREWORD

Just prior to the 1982 Annual Meeting of the European Thyroid Association in Brussels, a number of outstanding experts in the field of X-ray fluorescence gathered at the Academisch Ziekenhuis of the Free University of Brussels in a joint effort to more clearly define the actual place and value of the latest newcomer among the techniques available for the in vivo assessment of thyroid function. It is the merit of Prof. M. Jonckheer to have organised this meeting and to have made available the work presented there to a larger public in the form of this monograph. Both, the meeting and the written accounts thereof are greatly appreciated by all thyroidologists who care for properly defining the genuine value of X-Ray fluorescence in scientific research and in clinical management of thyroid disorder.

Three main conclusions can be drawn from the work presented :
1. X-ray fluorescence has become a safe, convenient and reliable tool for measuring intrathyroidal iodine stores in vivo with an inter-assay reproducibility estimated at roughly 10%
2. X-ray fluorescence, used by expert hands, is a highly interesting tool to follow changes of intrathyroidal iodine stores in time, subsequent e.g. to the exposure of the thyroid gland to excess iodine
3. In contrast, no definite place of X-ray fluorescence as a technique in routine assessment of thyroid disease is yet at the horizon

This latter conclusion may appear somewhat disappointing. However, it could be anticipated from the days the new technique had been created since it is well known that the total iodine content of the thyroid gland is barely correlated with its function. A small amount of highly iodinated thyroglobulin stored within follicles with highly active metabolism may well maintain hyperthyroidism, while large goiters in areas with poor iodine supply may still contain surprisingly large amounts of total iodine. Cold nodules of multinodular goiters often contain large iodine stores secluded from active metabolism. Moreover, it is only recently that knowledge is accumulated about the non-thyroglobulin-iodine which may amount to a large fraction of total thyroidal iodine in benign and malignant thyroid tissue. It is indeed one of the major shortcomings of X-ray fluorescence that it cannot distinguish the functionally important thyroglobulin from other fractions of intrathyroidal iodine. Against this background of thyroid physiology and pathophysiology, it is probably fair to conclude that the meeting has shown X-ray fluorescence to have come of age as a highly rewarding research tool but that its prospects for penetrating the daily routine work-up of thyroid disorders are rather dim.

Prof. H. STUDER
University Clinic
of Internal Medicine
Berne, Switserland.

## ACKNOWLEDGEMENTS

We want to thank Prof. C. Raynaud, President of the IIIrd World Congress of Nuclear Medicine, Paris, August 1982, who suggested us to organize a Post-Congress Meeting on X-Ray Fluorescence and the Thyroid.

This meeting took place in Brussels on September 4, 1982 and we were lucky on that day to find many experts in this field gathered together in lively discussions, among whom Drs P. Fragu (Paris), A. Magrini (Rome), H.W. Wahner (Rochester, USA), R. Leisner (Munchen), M.N. Maisey (London) and also S. Refetoff (Chicago), who took the chair in the afternoon. To all these participants goes our deep gratitude.

We are thankful to Dr P. Cox to have suggested the idea of this monograph, idea to which all participants of the meeting, as well as experts who could not attend it, agreed with enthousiasm. The book was conceived more as a state of the art monograph, rather than as true proceedings. A maximum of freedom was left to the different authors. It follows that some discrepancies and contradictions may be found but it was felt that this approach would be the most objective one, which would give the reader the best opportunity to make his own opinion about the subject.

Finally, the expert secreterial help of Mrs A. De Troyer is gratefully acknowledged.

The Editors.

Contributing Centers :

- Institut de Recherches de Radiobiologie Clinique INSERM
  Rue Camille Desmoulins - F-94805 Villejuif Cedex, France

  B. Aubert
  P. Fragu
  M. Schlumberger
  M. Tubiana

- Vanderbilt University Nashville, School of Medicine,
  Division of Radiological Sciences
  Tennessee 37232, U.S.A.

  J.A. Patton
  R.R. Price

- Guy's Hospital, Department of Nuclear Medicine
  St Thomas Street - London SE1 9RT, U.K.

  M.N. Maisey
  S.C. Ng Tang Fui

- IIa Cattedra di Fisica, Universita degli studi di Roma
  Citta Universitaria - I-00185 Roma, Italy

  S. Di Luzio
  G. Izzo
  A. Magrini
  P. Pavoni
  L. Raganella

- Mayo Clinic Department of Laboratory Medicine
  Rochester, Minnesota 55901, U.S.A.

  H.W. Wahner

- Radiologische Poliklinik der Universität München,
  Nuklearmedizinische Abteilung
  Ziemssenstrasse 1 - 8000 München 2, D.B.R.

  B. Leisner

- Akademisch Ziekenhuis - Vrije Universiteit Brussel,
  Dienst Radioisotopen
  Laarbeeklaan 101 - B-1090 Brussel, Belgium

  F. Deconinck
  M. Jonckheer

**PART I:** FUNDAMENTAL AND TECHNICAL ASPECTS

I  THEORETICAL BASES OF XRF

   F.Deconinck

1. INTRODUCTION

The process of exciting the electronic structure of stable elements by means of X- or gamma-rays to emit characteristic radiation is termed X-ray energy spectroscopy (XES), fluorescent excitation analysis (FEA), or X-ray fluorescence (XRF). When an element is exposed to X- or gamma-rays, the energy of which is higher than the binding energy of the K-shell (or L-shell) electrons in that element, vacancies can be created in that shell. That vacancy can be subsequently filled by an L-shell (or M-shell) electron . In this process, the atom can emit a photon with energy K (or L). The energy of this characteristic fluorescent radiation is unique to each element. It depends on the atomic number of the element and ranges from 1 to 100 keV (1 keV = $1,6.10^{-16}$ Joule). As the fluorescent excitation involves the K- or L-shells, XRF is not dependent on the chemical state of the element, and the number of characteristic photons emitted by a sample is proportional to the abundance of the element in the sample that is assayed (1,2,3).

In this chapter we will analyse the electronic structure of atoms, the different photon-matter interactions (with emphasis on those of interest in XRF) and the different mechanisms by which an excited atom can return to a stable electronic state.

## 2. PHYSICAL PRINCIPLES OF X-RAY FLUORESCENCE

### 2.1. <u>Electronic</u> <u>structure</u> <u>of</u> <u>the</u> <u>atom</u>

XRF is based on transitions of electrons within the atomic structure. Knowledge of the atomic structure is therefore essential for the understanding of XRF. The electronic structure of atoms depends on the number of protons Z in the nucleus and on the energetic state of the atom. We will assume that the atom is in its ground state. Mechanisms by which the atom is excited or deexcited will be discussed later. The correct description of the electronic structure requires the understanding of quantum mechanics. The property which is important for XRF is the distribution of the electrons on discrete shells around the nucleus. This property is described by the simplified Bohr model.

### 2.1.1. The Bohr Model

The electronic structure of the elements depends on the atomic number Z, which gives the number of protons in the nucleus, or the number of electrons around the nucleus. The electrons are bound to the positive nucleus by the attractive Coulomb force. The nuclear model of the atom proposed by Bohr results in a distribution of electrons around the nucleus on shells. The shells can be subdivided in subshells. Each electron, bound to the nucleus within a shell or subshell can be characterised by four numbers (n, l, m, s) which are its four quantum numbers. Due to the Pauli exclusion principle no two electrons can have the same set of quantum numbers (4,5).

The principal quantum number n=1, 2, ... defines the major shell. n=1 corresponds to the K-shell; n=2 to the L-shell etc... Each shell can be populated by a maximum of $2n^2$ electrons. The two K-shell electrons are most tightly bound to the nucleus. The next most tightly bound shell is the n=2 or L-shell which is composed of a maximum of 8 electrons on 4 subshells, defined by means of the orbital angular momentum $l = 0$ or 1 (there are n values of l for each n), its projection on an axis in space m (there are $2 l + 1$ values of m for each l), and the spin quantum number $(+ 1/2$ and $- 1/2)$. Similarly, the other shell and subshell configurations can be built up.

The binding of the electron decreases with increasing principal quantum number. When an electron of the K-shell is missing from the atom, the atom will be in its highest state of single electron excitation. The atom will return to a lower excitation state by filling the vacancy with an electron from a lighter bound shell. Electron transfers to vacant places must satisfy specific selection rules. Not all the transitions are allowed: transitions involving no change in orbital momentum are forbidden. The difference in energy between both shells can give rise to characteristic radiation. K X-ray lines correspond to the filling of a K-shell vacancy, L lines to a vacancy in one of the L-subshells, etc... In most XRF applications such as for the detection of I, the K X-rays will be used. For the assessment of heavy metals the L-lines can be choosen. The energy of the K- or L-lines is a function of the element, but not of the chemical state of the element which is influenced by the outer and not the inner electrons. The relative intensity of some lines can be deduced from the Greek characters following the X-ray designition, $\alpha$ being more intense than $\beta$ etc... The intensity of any given line will depend on the mode of deexcitation of the atom. This point will be discussed after the description of the photon matter interactions.

## 2.2. Photon-matter interactions

When a photon flux is directed towards a sample of matter, a number of photons will interact with the sample.

The number is a function of the energy of the photons E, the atomic number Z of the elements in the sample, its density $\rho$ (g/cm$^3$) and thickness x (cm). For a monochromatic X-ray beam, the intensity of the incident flux I(0) will decrease as a function of sample thickness according to

$$I(x) = I(0)e^{-\mu\rho x}$$

where $\mu$ represents the mass absorption coefficient. The mass absorption coefficient is a measure of the probability that the photons will interact with matter, regardless of the interaction mode (Figure 1).

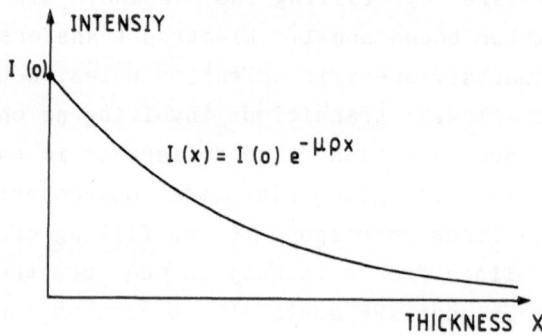

Figure 1. The absorption of monochromatic X-rays.

There are three primary modes of interaction :
- The photo-electric effect, on which XRF is based, and in which the original photon disappears by transferring all its energy to an electron.
- Scattering, which can be coherent (Rayleigh, Thomson) and in which the photon changes direction without energy loss, or incoherent (Compton) in which the photon changes direction with partial energy transfer to an electron.
- Pair production, in which an electron-positron pair is created. The probability for pair production is zero for photon energies less than 1 MeV, and will not be discussed here.

The relative importance of the different interaction modes is expressed by means of the cross section which describes the probability that an interaction will occur between the particle (here : photon) and the target (here : atom). The cross section is usually expressed in Barn/atom. 1 Barn = $10^{-28}$ $m^2$ (2,3,6,7,8).

2.2.1. The photo-electric effect

In the photo-electric effect, the energy of the incoming photon is totally transferred to an electron of the atom and the electron leaves the atom (Figure 2).

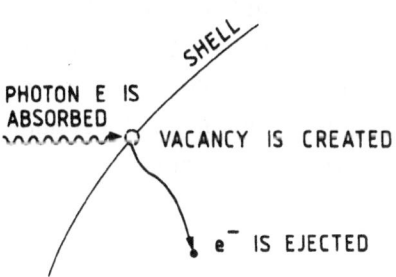

Figure 2. The photo-electric effect.

When a photon beam is directed at a sample, the probability for a photo-electric interaction is a function of the energy E of the photon and of the atomic number Z of the atoms in the sample. General trends are that the probability decreases as $E^{-3}$ and increases as $Z^4$. As long as the energy of an incoming photon is lower than the binding energy of the electron on its shell no photo-electric interaction can occur (for I, the K-shell binding energy is 33.164 keV). Once the photon energy exceeds the binding energy, the photon can transfer all its energy E to the electron. During the interaction the total energy and total momentum is conserved. To leave its shell the electron uses an amount of energy equal to its binding energy. The remainder is kinetic energy of the electron after the interaction. When the photon energy equals the binding energy of the electron, the photo electric cross section will increase abruptly. This discontinuous increase is called an absorption edge, and each shell or subshell has its associated absorption edge which is superposed on the general $E^{-3}$ trend (Figure 3).

Conservation of total momentum implies momentum transfer from the photon to the atom. This transfer is much more probable for tightly bound electrons. This means that the probability of a photo-electric interaction will be much higher for K-shell than for L- or M-shell electrons, provided the photon energy is sufficiently high. The cross section at the K edge will decrease with increasing Z, as the photon energy has to increase. However, at fixed energy the probability will be highest for high Z elements.

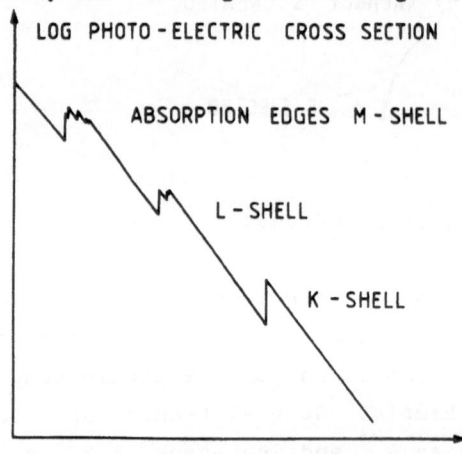

Figure 3. The photo-electric cross section and absorption edges.

## 2.2.2. Coherent Rayleigh scattering

When a photon beam passes through matter, photons can undergo scatter. In the interaction they change direction, with or without loss of energy. In coherent Rayleigh scattering there is no energy loss. The scattering mechanism can be visualised as follows : the incident wave of light induces an oscillation of the entire electronic structure of the atom. This oscillation reirradiates the incident radiation (Figure 4). The probability of this mode of scattering, which is well known for visible light, decreases with increasing energy (in the range of energies which is relevant to us) but increases with $Z^2$.

The coherent scattering is important in XRF because the coherent scatter peak will appear in the spectrum of the sample which is excited and can therefore be used for energy calibration of the spectrum. It is normally the peak in the spectrum with the highest energy.

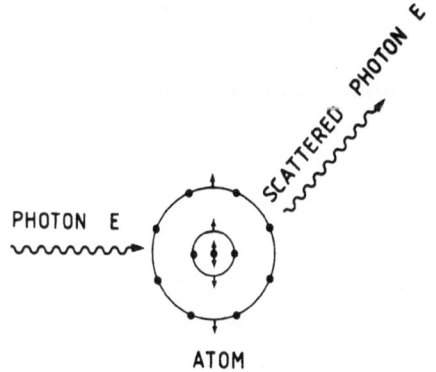

Figure 4. Coherent scattering.

2.2.3. Incoherent Compton scattering

In incoherent scattering the interaction can be visualised as the elastic collision of the incident photon with a single electron of the atom. The electron is supposed to be free. In an elastic collision, total energy and momentum are conserved. The photon transfers part of its energy and momentum to the electron. The incident photon changes direction and the electron gaines kinetic energy (Figure 5).

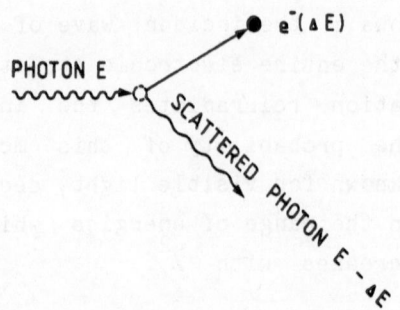

PHOTON E

e⁻(ΔE)

SCATTERED PHOTON E -ΔE

Figure 5. Incoherent scattering.

The photon scattering is not isotropic. Furthermore the scattered photon energy depends on the scatter angle and on the original photon energy. The Compton interaction describes the collision of the photon with a free, unbound electron at rest. This approximation (which is obviously incorrect in our case) yields good results because the probability of a Compton interaction becomes very small when the binding energy of the electron is comparable with the energy of the incoming photon. In the latter case the photo-electric interaction is most probable. The number of lightly bound electrons in an atom increases with Z. Therefore, the probability of a Compton interaction will also increase with Z. At energies above 1 MeV, the Compton interaction is dominant over the photo-electric effect. At energies under 100 keV, the photo-electric interaction is dominant for all elements with Z > 20. The Compton scattering results in a broad scatter peak with a mean energy which is lower than the incident photon energy. The energy shift increases with scatter angle, and with energy at fixed angle (at 90° the energy shift is 6.2 keV at 59.57 keV). For most energies used in XRF, the Compton peak is least intense at scatter angles of 90 to 100 degrees (7).

## 2.3. Deexcitation modes of the atom

When an atom is in an excited state because of the removal of an electron of an inner shell, and electrons (with the correct quantum numbers) are present on the less tightly bound shells or subshells, then the atom will return to a lower energetic state by filling the vacancy by one of its other electrons. The atom may deexcite (this is : transfer the energy liberated by the transfer of the electron from one state to a lower one) through the emission of a characteristic X-ray, through the emission of an Auger electron or by transfer of vacancies within a single shell. We will restrict ourselves to the first two mechanisms (2,3,6,7,8).

### 2.3.1.Characteristic radiation

When an atomic transition occurs, in which an electron transfer takes place from a less to a more tightly bound shell, the electron will decrease its total energy. Due to Planck's law ($\Delta E = h\nu$) the difference of the binding energy between the shells gives rise to a characteristic photon with an energy which is exactly the difference of the binding energies. These are the characteristic photons (Figure 6).

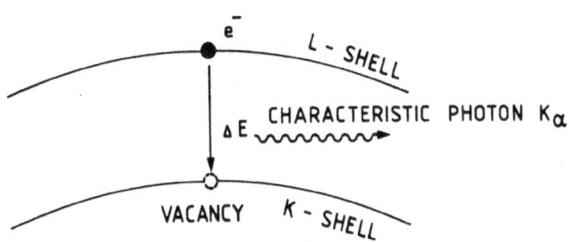

Figure 6. Characteristic radiation.

Due to the selection rules not all transitions are allowed, and the probability of each transition is different. Different probabilities give rise to different line intensities. For I the most intense lines are the $K_{\alpha 1}$ line (28.61 keV, relative intensity 100; corresponding to a L-K transition), the $K_{\alpha 2}$ line (28.315 keV, relative intensity 54 ; L-K transition), the $K_{\beta 1}$ line (32.289 keV, relative intensity 27.6; M-K transition) and the $K_{\beta 2}$ line (33.036 keV, relative intensity 5.4; N-K transition). Important for XRF is that the energy of the characteristic photons is specific to each element and not measurably dependent on the chemical state of the element.

## 2.3.2. Auger electrons - Fluorescent yield

The atom can also deexcite by transferring the vacancy to a higher shell, associated with the emission of an electron from the higher shell. The effect can be visualised as the reabsorption, internal to the atom, of the characteristic X-ray emitted during the transition.

If the atom can deexcite without emission of characteristic radiation, the yield of X-rays must be less than the number of vacancies formed. The probability of emission of an Auger electron decreases with increasing atomic number. For lighter elements (Z < 30), Auger electron emission is more probable than X-ray emission. The probability that a K-shell vacancy will be filled through a radiative transition, i.e. a characteristic X-ray is termed fluorescent yield. For I the fluorescent yield is 88 % (1).

## 3. THE XRF SPECTRUM

Shown in Figure 7 is the XRF spectrum obtained by irradiating a water solution containing I traces with Am-241 gamma rays (59.57 keV; a complete list of the Am-241 emission spectrum is found in reference 8. A 90° geometry between source-sample and detector was adopted. The detector used was a $1N_2$ cooled 80 mm$^2$ Si(Li) detector. The vertical axis represents the number of detected photons (linear scale) and the horizontal axis represents the photon energy in keV.

Four regions are characteristic to the spectrum :

region A corresponds mainly to Compton scatter in the detector

region B corresponds mainly to multiple scatter (in the detector and in the sample) and the characteristic I lines ($K_\alpha$, $K_\beta$)

region C corresponds to Compton scatter in the sample

region D corresponds to coherent scatter in the sample

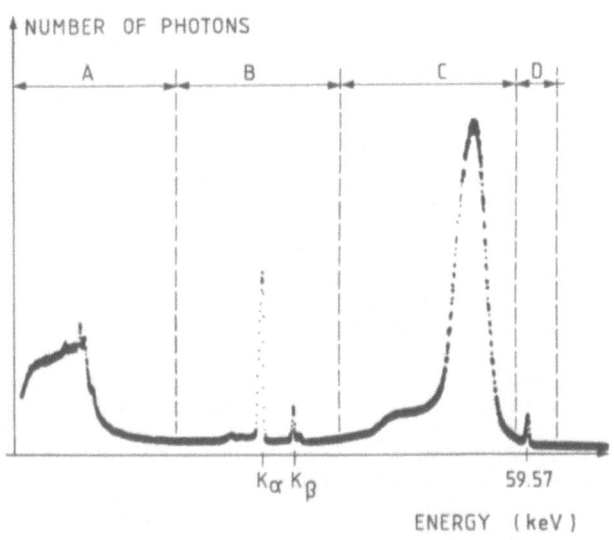

Figure 7. XRF spectrum of I in $H_2O$

region A is not used for XRF and only adds dead-time to the system

region B shows the characteristic I lines. $K_{\alpha 1}$ and $K_{\alpha 2}$ are not resolved. $K_{\beta 1}$ and $K_{\beta 2}$ are resolved and of much lower intensity than the $K_\alpha$ lines

To the left of the $K_\alpha$ lines, a small Am-241 line is seen (scatter of 26.36 keV line).

The background under the $K_\alpha$, $K_\beta$ lines should be substracted when quantification is reauired.

region C    shows the broad Compton scatter line, centered around 53 keV. The Compton scatter peak is broadened because of the range of scatter angles accepted by the source-sample-detector geometry.

In in-vivo XRF of the thyroid, the Compton scatter peak may overlap with the characteristic I lines.

region D    shows the coherent Rayleigh scatter in the sample. The energy of the line is 59.57 keV and can be used for calibration purposes.

## REFERENCES

01. Woldseth R. 1973. X-Ray Energy Spectrometry. Kevex Corporation, California, U.S.A.
02. Kaufman L., Price D. (Eds) 1979. Medical applications of fluorescent excitation analysis. CRC Press, Florida, U.S.A.
03. Hoffer P., Beck R., Gottschalk A. (Eds). 1971. The role of semiconductor detectors in the future of nuclear medicine. The Society of Nuclear Medicine, New York, U.S.A.
04. Herzberg G. Atomic spectra and atomic structure. Dover Publications, New York, U.S.A.
05. Woodgate G.K. Elementary atomic structure. McGraw-Hill, London, U.K.
06. Kaufman L., Price D. (Eds) 1973. Semiconductor detectors in medicine. U.S. Atomic Energy Commission, CONF-730321, Virginia, U.S.A.
07. Marmier P., Sheldon E. 1969. Physics of nuclei and particles. Academic Press, London, U.K.
08. Weast R.C. 1973. Handbook of chemistry and physics. CRC Press, Florida, U.S.A.

II INCIDENT SOURCES

B. AUBERT, P. FRAGU.

## INTRODUCTION

The nature of the element to be analysed by X-ray fluorescence (XRF) is the first criterion that determines the choice of the incident source. In fact we shall be including in the expression "incident source", not only the source of photons itself, but also its collimation and position relative to the detector, because of the considerable number of photons that are scattered by the Compton effect in function of the incident radiation energy and the angle between the axis of the photon beam and that of the detector.

In the general context of XRF application to study of the thyroid gland, we shall begin by discussing the physical problems of this application and, given these problems, the sources that are available ; we shall then describe the sources used in the in vitro analysis of thyroid tissues as well as in in vivo thyroid investigations involving quantification of stable iodine and/or the scanning of the distribution of this iodine ; finally, we shall conclude by studying in greater detail the sources used in XRF scanning.

## PHYSICAL PROBLEMS :

The phenomenon of XRF is based on the excitation of an atom by the photoelectric effect using a beam of photons ($\gamma$ or X-rays). The energy $E_0$ of these photons must be sufficiently high for an electron in the K, L,... shells to be ejected. If we call $W_K$, $W_L$,... the binding energy of the electrons in the K, L,... shells respectively, this should give $E_0 > W_K$ ($W_K > W_L > ...$). This relationship determines the choice of the source of photons with energy $E_0$, since $W_K$ is specific to any given element. After ejection of the electron from the K shell, a rearrangement of the electron layers takes place, which results in the emission of fluorescent photons with an energy that is specific to the atom being excited : these photons constitue a spectrum of $K_\alpha$, $K_\beta$ ... X-rays, such that : $E_{K_\alpha} = W_K - W_L$, $E_{K_\beta} = W_K - W_M$ ...

The same phenomenon existes for the other layers, but because of its energy and abundance, only the K shell is accepted for XRF analysis of the thyroid. In this analysis, iodine is the element that is excited. Table 1 sets out some of the physical properties of this element. Fig. 1 shows that for this element the K shell fluorescent yield is high : 88.2 %.

Table 1. Some physical characteristics of iodine.

| Z | $W_K$ | $E_{K\alpha}$ | $E_{K\beta}$ |
|---|---|---|---|
| 53 | 33.2 keV | 28.5 keV | 32.6 keV |

The intensity of fluorescence is a function of the probability of a photo-electric effect, and since this is proportional to $E_0^{-3}$, it decreases rapidly as $E_0$ increases. Fig. 2 illustrates this decrease, if the photo-electric effect probability for $E_0$ = 35 keV is normalised to 100 %. There is therefore an advantage in using a source with an excitation energy $E_0$ as close as possible to the value of $W_K$, since in conditions of identical photon flux, the closer $E_0$ to $W_K$, the higher the fluorescent signal. This fact is weighted, however, by two physical phenomenon : the Compton scattered photons which become all the more numerous in the $K_\alpha$ ray as $E_0$ approaches $W_K$, and the tissue attenuation effect on incident photons which is all the greater as $E_0$ approaches $W_K$.

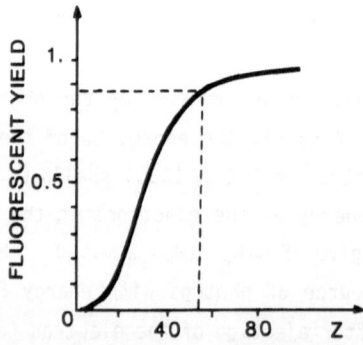

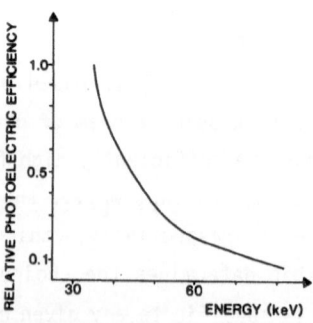

Figure 1 :
K-X ray fluorescent yield versus atomic number Z. In the case of iodine Z = 53 and fluorescent yield 88.2 %.

Figure 2 :
Variation of the relative photo-electric efficiency versus the energy of the K iodine discontinuity. Efficiency = 1 when the energy = 35 keV.

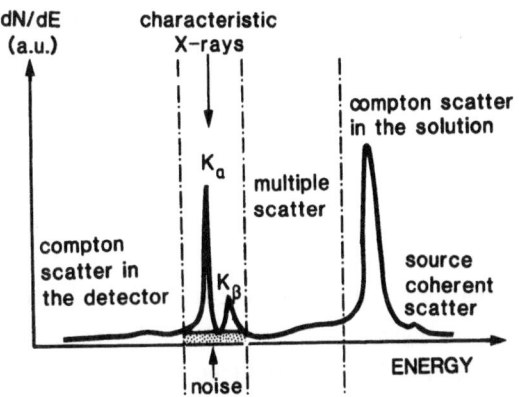

Figure 3 :
XRF spectrum obtained on an iodine solution with an americium 241 source (1).

Fig. 3 shows a spectrum of XRF obtained by the scattering of americium 241 photons on a solution of iodine (1). On this spectrum can be seen the peaks that are charactetistics of iodine (the $K_\alpha$ and $K_\beta$ peaks), the source coherent scattering peak, the single Compton scattering peak in the solution, the region of multiple scattering in this solution and the scattering region in the detector. The photons detected after single Compton scattering in tissue have an energy $E_s$ governed by the relationship :

$$ E_s = \frac{E_o}{1 + \dfrac{E_o}{m_o c^2} (1 - \cos \theta )} $$

where $\theta$ is the scattering angle fixed by the angle of the incident beam axis with the axis of the detector. The particularly interesting case is that in which

$$ E_s = E_{K\alpha} = 28.5 \text{ keV}. $$

Table 2 gives, for different values of $\theta$, the values of $E_o$ for which the single scattering peak corresponds to the iodine $K_\alpha$ X-ray (28.5 keV). The table shows that no source with an energy greater than $W_K$ can have its single scattering peak coinciding with the $K_\alpha$ X-ray, even though the width of this peak can vary with the collimation system being used and $K_\alpha$ X-ray detection is generally carried out between 27.5 and 29.5 keV.

<u>Table 2</u> : Value of photon incident energy $E_0$ versus scattering angle giving scattering energy $E_s = E_{K_\alpha} = 28.5$ keV

| Scattering angle θ (deg.) | 90 | 120 | 150 |
|---|---|---|---|
| Incident energy $E_0$ (keV) | 30.2 | 31.1 | 31.8 |

    Fig. 4 shows the variation of the water attenuation coefficient (water being similar from this point of view to thyroid and extra-thyroid tissue) in function of energy in the range 30 - 100 keV. The thyroid lies from 0 to 50 mm under the skin, and thus we have set out in Fig. 5 the transmission of a photon beam through 3 tissues thicknesses : 10, 20 and 50 mm, each one of there curves being normalized against a standard value for 35 keV.

    If Figures 2 and 5 are compared, it can be seen that between 35 and 60 keV, the probability of photo-electric effect drops from 100 % to 20 %, whereas beam transmission at a thickness of 50 mm rises, respectively, from 100 % to 146 %. Thus overall, considering the intensity of the fluorescent signal, it is better to work with values for $E_0$ that are close to $W_K$.

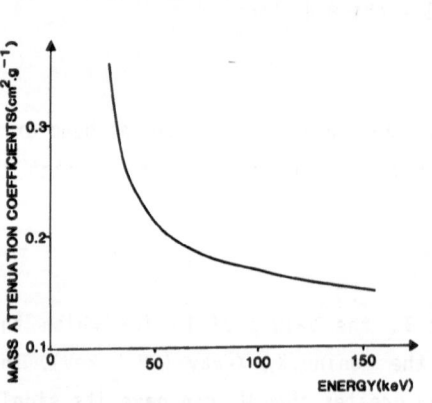

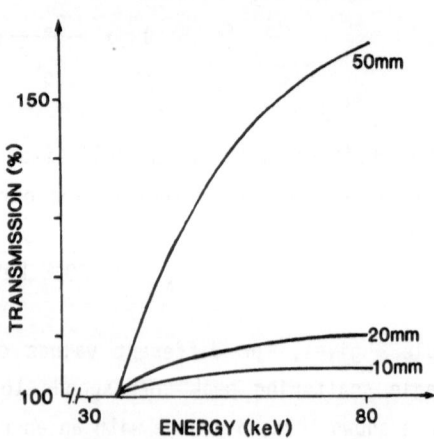

<u>Figure 4</u> :
Mass attenuation coefficient in the water versus energy.

<u>Figure 5</u> :
Transmission of a photon beam versus energy through 3 tissues of different thickness : 10,20,50 mm. Each curve is normalized at 35 keV.

## AVAILABLE SOURCES

It follows that the "ideal" source for the excitation of iodine should possess the following features :

- it should emit a photon beam with an energy $E_o$ greater than, but very close to $W_K$ (33.2 keV) ;
- it should have a very long an even "infinite" half-life ;
- it should have a high specific activity so as to give a beam that is as narrow as possible (1 to 2 mm).

Table 3 lists the radioactive sources giving out gamma rays with an energy ranging between $W_K$ and approximately 100 keV and with a sufficiently long half-life ($>$100 days) (2).

Table 3 : Main characteristics of radionuclides that can be used as incident sources for XRF thyroid analysis.

| Radionuclide | Half-life | $\gamma$ ray energy[+] keV | Emission % |
|---|---|---|---|
| $^{109}_{48}Cd$ | 450 d. | 88.036 | 3.7 |
| $^{155}_{63}Eu$ | 1.81 y. | 60.07 | 2.8 |
| | | 86.60 | 72.4 |
| | | 105.36 | 48.2 |
| $^{153}_{64}Gd$ | 242 d. | 103.18 | 100 |
| | | 97.43 | 132 |
| | | 69.68 | 11 |
| $^{159}_{66}Dy$ | 144 d. | 58.0 | 4 |
| $^{170}_{69}Tm$ | 128.6 d. | 84.262 | 3.4 |
| $^{241}_{95}Am$ | 458 y. | 59.57 | 36 |

[+] only when % emission $> 1$

data from : Handbook of Chemistry and Physics, 56th edition, 1975-6, CRCB.

A look at the table shows that none of the available sources correspond to the "ideal" ; when the energy is close to $W_K$, the half-life is among the shortest ($^{159}$Dy), and when the half-life is "infinity", the energy is much less suitable ($^{241}$Am).

To these $\gamma$ ray emitters must be added the X-ray generator. This apparatus gives a narrow photon beam with an adjustable intensity greater than that delivered by a radioactive source. By being able to adjust the high voltage and the filter system, the spectrum of X-ray beam can be optimised in rela- tion to the XRF signal and the energy radiation components that are lower than $W_K$ can be suppressed (these only increase the tissue dose and spoil the fluorescent signal to noise ratio in the $K_\alpha$ region).

## EXISTING SYSTEMS

Table 4 sets out the features of the majority of XRF equipment used for the in vitro or in vivo study of the thyroid. The features listed are only those that concern excitation, i.e. the radiation source (nature and activi- ty), the collimation system used for this source and the scattering angle (between the axis of the photon beam and the axis of detection) ; the table does not deal with any features of the detector or the electronic.

When Tables 3 and 4 are compared, it can be seen that out of the 7 sources that are theoretically available, only two are actually used in practice : americium 241 and the X-ray tube. The dysprosium 159 that Hoffer used in his early studies (11) was rapidly replaced by americium 241 on account of its price and short half-life.

Our own group used a thulium 170 source in 1974. The advantage of this source over americium 241 was a higher specific activity (222 GBq (6 Ci)) in a 4x4x4 mm$^3$ volume) and the fact that it was available in quantities of 2220 GBq (60 Ci) (21). However, its relatively short half-life (129 days) and the presence of photons with an energy ranging from 200 keV to several MeV which made heavy shielding necessary, and spoiled the fluorescent signal to noise ration, led us to abandon use of this source.

Comparison of radiation sources is therefore exclusively between ameri- cium 241 and the X-ray tube.

| REFERENCE | APPLICATION(+) | SOURCE | SOURCE COLLIMATOR | SCATTERING ANGLE |
|---|---|---|---|---|
| Le Blanc (1974) (3) | "in vitro" | 241Am (3,7 GBq) | collimated | 150° |
| Sikanen (1976) (4) | "in vitro" | 241Am (18.5 GBq)+cible Ce | cylindrical hole( 10mm-L:40mm) | 135° |
| Tadros (1981) (5) | "in vitro" | 241Am (11.1 GBq) | collimated | 90° |
| Kaufman (1973) (6) | "in vivo"I.Q. | 241Am (37 MBq) | cylindrical hole | 135° |
| Pavoni (1976) (7) | "in vivo"I.Q. | 241Am (2 x 1.7 GBq) | cylindrical hole ( 3,3mm-L:11mm) | 130° |
| Gollnick (1978) (8) | "in vivo"I.Q. | 241Am (?) | wide angle collimator |  |
| Imamura (1979) (9) | "in vivo"I.Q. | 241Am (1.11 GBq) | wide angle collimator |  |
| Maisey (1982) (10) | "in vivo"I.Q. | 241Am (1.11 GBq) | tapered hole | 60° |
| Hoffer (1968) (11) | "in vivo"I.D. | 159Dy (2x11.1 MBq) | collimated | 120° |
| Hoffer (1969) (12) | "in vivo"I.D. | 241Am (1.11 GBq) | tapered hole | 165° |
| Hoffer (1971) (13) | "in vivo"ID+IQ | 241Am (3x185 GBq) | collimated | 140° |
| Brill (1974) (14) | "in vivo"ID+IQ | 241Am (16x37 GBq) | tapered hole | 150° |
| Munkner (1974) (15) | "in vivo"ID+IQ | 241Am (1x370 GBq) | 253 hole double focusing collimator | 132° |
| Palmer (1976) (16) | "in vivo"ID+IQ | 241Am (1x370 GBq) | 57 hole double focusing collimator | 132° |
| Gillin (1977) (17) | "in vivo"ID+IQ | 241Am (20x37 GBq) | tapered hole | 150° |
| Esser (1977) (18) | "in vivo"I.D. | Xrays (80kV-0.5mA) | cylindrical hole($\emptyset$1,6mm-L=25,4mm) | 150° |
| Johnson (1979) (19) | " | " | " |  |
| Aubert (1977) (20) | "in vivo"ID+IQ | Xrays (80kV-4mA) | cylindrical hole($\emptyset$1,5mm-L=50mm) | 152° |

(+)I.Q. : iodine          I.D. : iodine distribution

TABLE 4

Characteristics of incident sources used in XRF systems for _in vitro_ and _in vivo_ thyroid study

## COMPARISON BETWEEN [241]Am AND THE X-RAY TUBE

The type of application for which the XRF equipment is required is the first step in choosing a radiation source.

For a system intended to be used for in vitro or in vivo quantification of intra-thyroidal iodine or for a dynamic study that does not involve realizing an image of the iodine distribution, the source is not finely collimated nor is the time taken by the investigation a major consideration. In such conditions, an [241]Am source of around 1 gigabequerel or several dozen gigabequerels (several dozen to several hundred mCi) is sufficient. In contrast, for an XRF system destined to show the distribution of intra-thyroidal iodine, a high photon flux must be available, together with a reasonable examination time ($\simeq 15$ min). Furthermore, the beam must be finely collimated to give good spatial resolution. Only an X-ray tube or an americium 241 source of several dozen gigabequerels (several curies) is enough to meet these requirements. The comparison between these two radiation sources really therefore concerns :
    - the quality and quantity of the photon flux available.
    - the efficiency of these photons in relation to the phenomenon of [127]I XRF ;
    - the fluorescent signal to noise ratio (S/N) in the $K_\alpha$ peak region ;
    - the cost and the auxiliary equipement required for each of these sources.

The incident source spectrum
-----------------------------

The monochromatic radiation of [241]Am contrasts with the polychromatic spectrum given out by an X-ray tube. In fact, the quality of the latter spectrum depends on the high voltage used and the X-ray tube filter system (its own filter + any additional filter). Given the energies necessary ($>W_K$), the high voltage must be no higher than 100 kV and even less. On Esser's system (18), as on our own (20), the high voltage equals 80 kV. In our own case, this limitation is imposed on us by the generator and type of tube used : a tungsten anode mammography tube, with a thin beryllium window. Esser (18) uses the same type of tube with a 0.75 mm Be window. This filter is not sufficient to lower the dose received by the patient (suppression of components with an energy lower than $W_K$) or to improve the S/N ratio. Additional filtering is therefore provided.

In Fig. 6, the fluorescent spectrum obtained by exciting a thyroid phantom containing a 2 mg/ml iodine solution placed under 20 mm water can be compared for 4 different additional filter thicknesses (0.5, 1.0, 1.5 and 2.0 mm copper). The spectrum at 0.5 mm filter thickness is clearly not being filtered enough, since a background noise can be seen that is far higher than in the other 3 spectra. Though it is only later that we shall be dealing quantitatively with the problem of the S/N ratio, it is worth noting that on the two systems using an X-ray tube, additional filtering is made up of 2 mm Cu + 1 mm Al in Esser's case (18) and 1 mm Cu in our own (20).

Given the foregoing physical considerations, it can already be seen that the features of the $^{241}$Am spectrum mean that energy is not being adapted in the best possible way to XRF, but on the other hand that background noise due to single Compton scattering in the $K_\alpha$ region is zero (scattering energy = 49 keV, for a scattering angle of 150°). In contrast, the photon spectrum given out by the X-ray tube is more effective from the iodine XRF point of view because of the components lying just above the value for $W_K$, but this greater effectiveness is achieved to the detriment of noise in the $K_\alpha$ region.

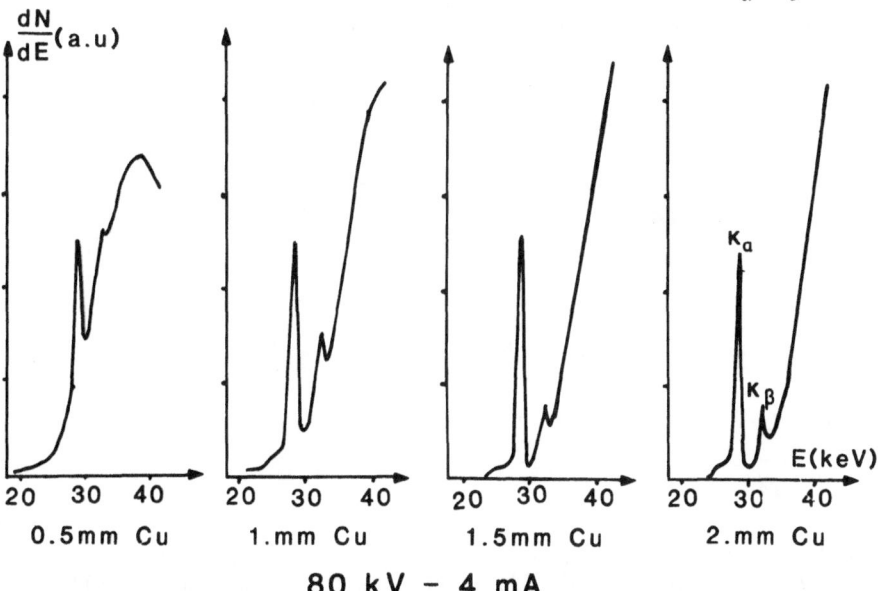

**80 kV - 4 mA**

Figure 6 : Fluorescent spectra obtained by exciting a thyroid phantom containing a 2 mg/ml iodine solution when 4 additional filters of different thickness of copper (0.5, 1.0, 1.5 and 2.0 mm) are used.

Collimation
-----------

In XRF thyroid imaging systems using $^{241}$Am, two basic geometric types are offered on the most recent models :
- one with a single 370 GBq (10 Ci) source with a 57- (16) or a 253- (15) hole collimator providing dual focussing of the incident beam at approximately 60 mm from the source collimator. Fig. 7 A is a diagram of such a system in which the axis of the detector meets the axis of the photon beam, at an angle of approximately 48° ;
- the other geometric arrangement is made up to several 37 GBq (1 Ci) source positioned on a circle, in a lead container, around the detector (Fig. 7 B). Each source is focused by a tapered hole, and the axes meet 45 mm from the collimator. The angle between the axis of the detector and that of the photon beam of each source is 30°. This multi-hole collimation in the case of a single source, or concentric distribution for several sources, is made necessary by the size of the $^{241}$Am sources : for a 37 GBq (1 Ci) source the active diameter is 25 mm (22). For an X-ray tube, it is so small (13 mm x 3 mm) that a single cylindrical collimator is sufficient. On Johnson's apparatus (19), it is 25.4 mm long and 1.6 mm wide, whereas on our own (23), the dimensions are 50 mm and 1.5 mm respectively (Fig. 8).

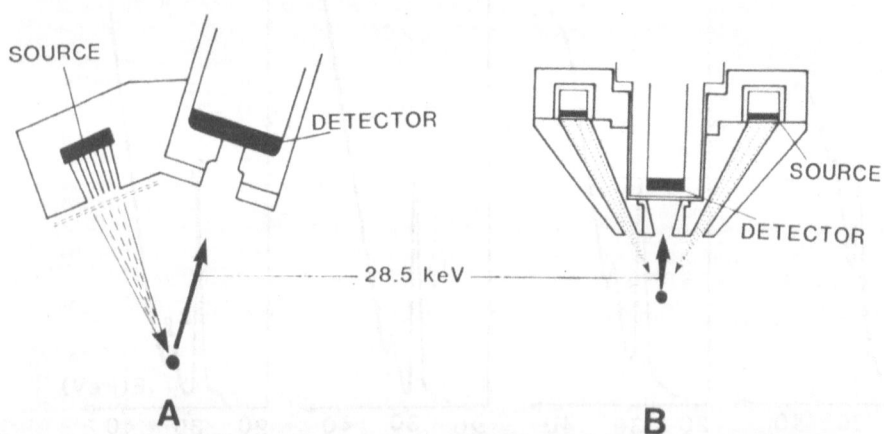

Figure 7: Fluorescent scanning systems with $^{241}$Am incident source.
         A : a single 370 GBq source with a multihole collimator (13),(15),(16).
         B : arrangement of several 37 GBq sources positionned on a circle around the detector (14), (17).

The angle of the axis of the X-ray beam with that of the detector is 30° in Johnson's system and 28° in our own.

Thus in practice, if the width of the photon beam is expressed by the full width a half maximum (FWHM) of the response to a line filled with iodine and placed in the focal plane, the values obtained with $^{241}$Am source systems are higher than those obtained with X-ray tube systems (Table 5).

Fluorescent signal to noise ratio
---------------------------------

This ratio expresses the fluorescent signal S picked up in the $K_\alpha$ peak region on a thyroid phantom of given iodine concentration in function of the signal N obtained in the $K_\alpha$ peak region in the absence of iodine.

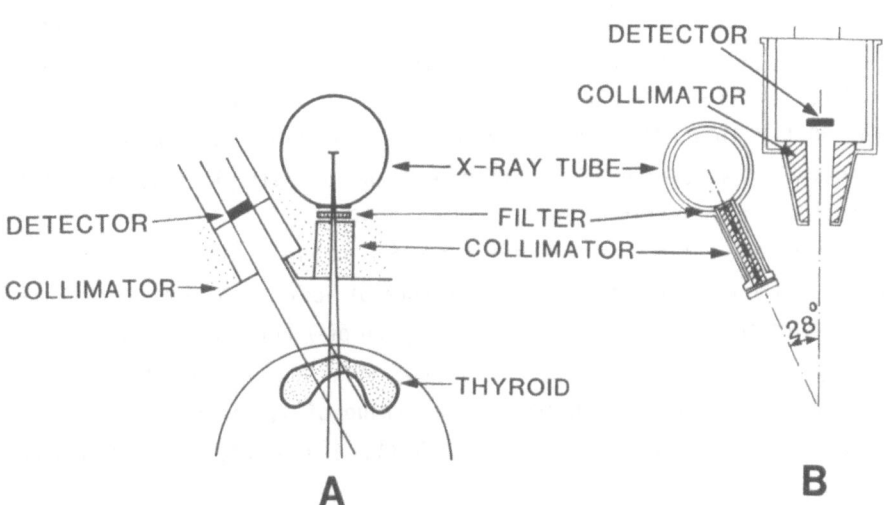

Figure 8 : Fluorescent scanning systems with an X-ray tube incident source
A : Johnson's equipment (18), (19)          B : Aubert's equipment (20).

Table 5 : Width of the radiation source beam expressed as the full width at half maximum (FWHM) of the response to an iodine line in the focal plane for some XRF thyroid imaging systems.

| RADIATION SOURCE | FWHM (mm) |
|---|---|
| $^{241}$Am      1 x 370 GBq (10 Ci) collimator : 57 holes (16) | 7.5 |
| $^{241}$Am      1 x 370 GBq (10 Ci) collimator : 253 holes (15) | 7.0 |
| $^{241}$Am      20 x 37 GBq (1 Ci) collimator : tapered hole (17) | 7.0 |
| X-ray tube (18) collimator : L = 25.4 mm, $\phi$ = 1.6 mm | 4.6 |
| X-ray tube (20) collimator : L = 50 mm,   $\phi$ = 1.5 mm | 3.0 |

This S/N ratio obviously depends on the detector energy resolution, the setting of the single channel analyser and on the radiation source spectrum. It is this last point that concern us.

It can be seen from Table 2 that, where the energy of $^{241}$Am is concerned, only multiple scattering in the irradiated tissue is a cause of noise in the K  region. As for the X-ray tube, given that its spectrum stretches from between 30 keV to 80-100 keV, noise is the sum of single scattering for components with an energy around 30-35 keV and of multiple scattering for components of higher energy.

Table 6 sets out for each of the 4 spectra of Fig. 6 the values of S + N (integral of the $K_\alpha$ peak region in the presence of iodine), N (integral of the $K_\alpha$ peak region in the absence of iodine), S/N and of T (time necessary for S to reach 100,000 imps). The attenuation of the X-ray beam can be evaluated in function of the filter by considering the value of T, since all the other parameters are identical (high voltage 80 kV, I = 4 mA, 2 mg/ml iodine solution).

A clear improvement (by a factor of 4.4) can be seen in the S/N ratio when one goes from 0.5 to 1 mm Cu. This improvement is maintained when filter thickness increases. However, it obviously diminishes the flux of photons. Therefore, taking the results obtained with 1 mm Cu as our reference point, if

Table 6 : Influence of Cu filter thickness on the value of the signal (S) to noise (N) ratio in the $K_\alpha$ peak region and on the time necessary to get S = 100,000 imps. Data were obtained with the X-ray tube operating at 80 kV and 4 mA and using a 2 mg/ml iodine solution.

| Filter (mm Cu) | 0.5 | 1.0 | 1.5 | 2.0 |
|---|---|---|---|---|
| Signal+Noise (imps) | 492,000 | 100,000 | 29,600 | 14,200 |
| Noise (imps) | 271,700 | 22,000 | 4,400 | 1,700 |
| S/N | 0.81 | 3.55 | 5.72 | 7.35 |
| Time (s) for S = 100,000 imps | 336 | 950 | 2783 | 5962 |

we wish to keep the same signal S for any given concentration of iodine, either the mA have to be increased, or else scanning has to be slowed. Thus for 1.5 mm, a gain of a factor of 1.6 in the S/N ratio is compensated for by a factor of 3 in signal acquisition time or mA. These values are 2.1 and 6.3 respectively for 2 mm Cu.

Since the parameters 4 mA and 15 min scanning are those which, with 1 mm Cu, mean that only 0.4 m Gy (40 mrad) will be delivered to the patient's skin, at the same time as detecting 379 imps/mg iodine, if we wish to maintain scanning time, and the value of signal S all the same, then we must work at 12 mA for 1.5 mm Cu and at 25 mA for 2 mm Cu. With the tube's permissible maximum being 15 mA, it is impossible to use 2 mm Cu and a little awkward to work at such a high intensity for 1.5 mm Cu, furthermore patient irradiation increases.

To compare S/N ratios with [241]Am and X-rays, the same detection and electronics system must be used, as well as the same spectrometric settings (Fig. 9). Under these conditions, we were able to compare a 74 GBq (2 Ci) [241]Am source collimated by 19 converging holes and delivering a beam with a FWHM of 6 mm, with an X-ray tube working at 80 kV - 4 mA filtered by 1 mm Cu and collimated by a 1.5 mm cylindrical tube. In addition, the dose D delivered to the point of convergence between the two axes (source and detector) in the air was measured using thermoluminescent dosimeters. We were thus able to express the S/D ratio, which gives the value of the fluorescent signal detected per gray delivered. This ratio should be maximum for any given system.

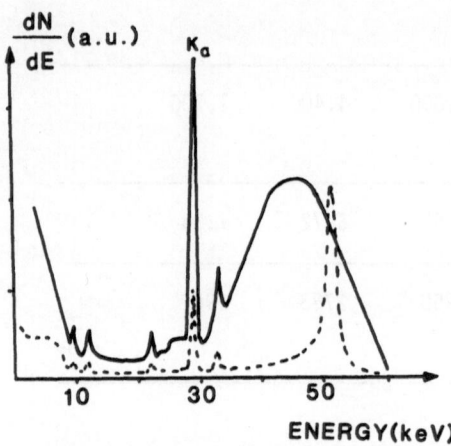

Figure 9
Spectra obtained after scattering on an iodine solution in the case of an X-ray tube (——) and in the case of a 241Am source (----). The detector, the electronic material and the spectrometric settings are the same in both cases.

Table 7 gives these S, N, S/N, D and S/D values for the $^{241}$Am source and the X-ray tube placed in the same configuration with the same detector, with the same electronics and settings.

Table 7 : Comparison of ratio S (XRF signal) to N (noise) and ratio S to D (dose at focal plane) for 241Am and X-ray tube as incident source. Electronic, spectrometric and detector settings are the same for both sources.

| Radiation source | Signal (imps/s) | Noise (imps/s) | S/N | Dose rate (cGy/h) | S/D (imps/Gy) |
|---|---|---|---|---|---|
| $^{241}$Am 74 GBq (2 Ci) | 0.43 | 0.31 | 1.38 | 0.244 | 63.4 |
| X-ray tube 80 kV - 4 mA ($\phi$ = 1.5 mm) filter : 1 mm Cu | 4.3 | 2.8 | 1.56 | 1.62 | 96.0 |

Tables 6 and 7 are not directly comparable as the conditions of measurement and some elements in the measurement system are different.

Cost and auxiliary equipement
-----------------------------

The disadvantages of $^{241}$Am sources are simply those of storing a source with a high activity (several hundred GBq) and a very long half-life (450 years). Once the source has been acquired, nothing further need interrupt its use. At the present time, the 20 sources are available for approx. $25,000 (without tax).

As for X-ray tubes, besides their bulkiness as far as the excitation-detection systems is concerned, water cooling must be provided, as well as a site for the generator, and also cables linking the generator to the tube. In addition, if theoretically the tube has an "infinite" half-life, in fact it has to be replaced after several years.

The cost of the generator + tube + X-ray tube housing is approximately $18,000 (without tax). The cost of tube replacement is approximately $1500 (without tax).

CONCLUSION

Though its radiation (59.5 keV) is rather far removed from the value of the binding energy of the iodine K shell (33.2 keV), $^{241}$Am is the source of choice for an XRF system intended for the in vitro or in vivo quantification of thyroid iodine. For in vitro work, acquisition time is not a problem and as for in vivo studies, which can be carried out with wide collimation (the entire thyroid gland is excited simultaneously by the photon beam), the signal obtained by a source of 37 GBq (1 Ci) or less is sufficient.

When XRF is being used to obtain an image of the intra-thyroid distribution of stable iodine, examination time must be taken into account (it should not exceed 15 mn), and also the signal, which must be sufficiently strong. It then becomes necessary to use $^{241}$Am sources with an activity as high as 740 GBq (20 Ci). In such cases, an alternative does exist, which is to use an X-ray tube as a source of excitation. Proper choice of high voltage, mA, filtering and collimation give a considerable photon flux with a spectrum ranging from approximately 30 keV to 80 keV and results in a higher fluorescent yield than with $^{241}$Am. This gain in yield compensates for the increased multiple scattering in the $K_\alpha$ peak region.

REFERENCES

1. Allemand R. 1978. L'instrumentation pour la fluorescenceX. Symposium sur les applications de la fluorescence X in vitro en biologie et en médecine. Grenoble p. 83-99.

2. Allemand R, Benabib A, Hellouin Y, Laval M. 1973. Une application des détecteurs semi-conducteurs en médecine nucléaire, la fluorescence X in vivo. Note technique LETI/MCTE 924.

3. Le Blanc AD, Bell RL, Johnson PC. 1974. Measurement of $^{127}$I concentration in thyroid tissue by X-ray fluorescence. J. Nucl. Med. 14:816-819.

4. Sikanen P, Olkkonen H, Patomäki L. 1976. A technique for the measurement of stable iodine in tissues using X-ray fluorescence and Compton scattering. Invest. Radiol. 11:60-62.

5. Tadros TG, Maisey MN, Ng Tang Fui SC, Turner PC. 1981. The iodine concentration in begnin and malignant thyroid nodules measured by X-ray fluorescence. Br. J. Radiol. 54:626-629.

6. Kaufman L, Shames D, Powell M. 1973. An absorption correction technique for in vivo iodine quantitation by fluorescent excitation. Invest. Radiol. 8:167-169.

7. Pavoni P, Frazolli FV, Magrini A. 1976. Radioisotope X-ray fluorescence technique in the dynamic study of thyroid behaviour under iodine load. Eur. J. Nucl. Med. 1:117-122.

8. Gollnick DA, Greenfield MA. 1978. The in vivo measurement of the total iodine content of the thyroid gland by X-ray fluorescence. Radiology 126:197-200.

9. Imamura K, Sasaki Y, Sekita N, Someya K, Fujii M. 1979. Quantitative in vivo measurement of thyroidal iodine content by static X-ray fluorescent technique : some preliminary clinical observations. Invest. Radiol. 14:316-322.

10. Maisey MN, Ng Tang Fui SC. 1982. The differenciation between benign and malignant thyroid nodules using X-ray fluorescence with a stationary single detector. Nuclear Medicine and Biology. (Proc. of the Third World Congress of Nuclear Medicine and Biology). C. Raynaud Editor. Pergamon Press, Paris, 87-89.

11. Hoffer PB, Jones WB, Crawford RB, Beck R., Gottschalk A. 1968. Fluorescent thyroid scanning : a new method of imaging the thyroid. Radiology 90:342-344.

12. Hoffer PB, Charleston DB, Beck RN, Gottschalk A. 1969. Fluorescent scanning : a new investigative technique. In : Medical Radioisotope Scintigraphy. I.A.E.A., Vienna 1:261-271.

13. Hoffer PB, Gottschalk A. 1971. Fluorescent thyroid scanning : scanning without radioisotopes. Radiology 99:117-123.

14. Brill AB, Patton JA, Hollifield J. 1974. Thyroid fluorescent scanning. In : Proceedings of a symposium on thyroid and endocrine system investigations with radionuclides. Miami. Chap. 6.

15. Munkner T. 1974. Iodine fluorescent scintigraphy. In : XVI Colloque de Médecine Nucléaire de Langue Française, Clermont Ferrand.

16. Palmer DW, Deconinck F, Swann SJ, Okerlund M, Kaufman L., Hoffer PB. 1976. Low cost intrathyroidal iodine quantification with a fluorescent scanner. Radiology 119:733-735.

17. Gillin MT, Thrall JH, Corcoran RJ, Johnson MC.1977. Evaluation of a thyroid fluorescent scanning system of concentric source-detector design. J. Nucl. Med. 18:163-167.

18. Esser PD, Lister DB. 1977. A new apparatus for fluorescent scanning : a moving X-ray tube. abst. J. Nucl. Med. 18:640.

19. Johnson PM, Esser PD, Lister DB. 1979. Fluorescent thyroid imaging : clinical evaluation of an alternative instrument. Radiology. 130:219-222.

20. Aubert B, Di Paola M, Laval M, Allemand R, Fragu P, Tubiana M. 1977. Fluorescence X par excitation à l'aide d'un générateur de rayons X. Application à la thyroïde. In : XVIII Colloque de Médecine Nucléaire de Langue Française, Reims.

21. Laval M. Personnal Communication.

22. The Radiochemical Centre Amersham (1981). Catalogue RS 16-4 : 12.

23. Aubert B, Fragu P, Di Paola M, Rougier P, Tubiana M. 1981. Application of X-ray fluorescence to the study of iodine distribution and content in the thyroid. Eur. J. Nucl. Med. 6:407-410.

# III DETECTION SYSTEMS FOR XRF STUDIES OF THE THYROID

JAMES A. PATTON and RONALD R. PRICE

X-ray fluorescence (XRF) applications require detectors with ultra-high energy resolution. The primary detectors fulfilling this requirement that are currently available are semiconductor radiation detectors. These devices are often referred to as solid state detectors because their origin lies in the development of materials for transistor technology. They are the detectors of choice for virtually all work in nuclear spectroscopy.

Before elaborating on the basics of semiconductor detector technology, a brief review of the interactions of electromagnetic radiation with matter is appropriate to provide for a better understanding of their operation. Most XRF applications involve the detection of x-rays of energy less than 50 KeV (iodine $K_\alpha$ x-ray energies are about 28.5 KeV). In this energy range the two primary photon interactions are photoelectric absorption and Compton scattering.

Photoelectric absorption in a material involves the absorption of the incident photon by an inner shell electron of an atom. The electron (called the photoelectron) is then ejected from the atom with an energy equal to the incident photon energy minus the binding energy of the electron in its shell. The atom is then left in an ionized and excited state. It de-excites by outer shell electrons dropping down to fill the inner shell vacancies with the excess energy being released in the form of characteristic radiation (x-rays or Auger electrons). This is low energy radiation and is generally absorbed by the surrounding medium.

Compton scattering is the process whereby a photon interacts with a loosely bound electron with the electron receiving some of the energy of the photon. The electron recoils at an angle $\theta$ with respect to the direction of travel of the incident photon. The photon also has its direction of travel altered by some angle $\phi$. The amount of energy transferred to the electron depends on the angle of scattering of the photon $\phi$. The scattered photon leaves the point of interaction with reduced energy and may then undergo another Compton interaction or photoelectric absorption.

Thus the result of photoelectric absorption and Compton scattering of photons is the creation of one or more ion pairs (the freed electron carrying off part of the energy of the incident photon and the atom minus one electron). If the characteristic radiation resulting from photoelectric absorption and the scattered photon from Compton scattering undergo subsequent interactions in the material, the total interaction is classified as a total absorption event with the energies of the positive and negative ions being a measure of the incident photon energy. The electrons produced in these interactions possess sufficient energy to interact with other electrons to produce secondary ionizations (i.e., additional ion pairs). The total number of ion pairs produced then provides a mechanism for the detection of the incident photon and a measurement of its energy.

This concept forms the basis for the operation of gas-type ionization detectors (ionization chambers, proportional counters, and Geiger Muller counters) as illustrated in Figure 1. Ionization detectors, as the name implies, make use of the direct ionization of a sensitive volume of gas to measure radiation. A gas-filled volume is placed between two electrodes, one connected to the positive side of a d.c. power supply such as a battery and the other connected to the negative side. Thus, a potential difference is established between the two plates. A sensitive device for measuring current flow is also placed in the circuit. Under normal conditions with no radiation present, there is no flow of current between the electrodes and the current meter registers zero. However, when radiation passes through the sensitive volume, it interacts with the gas by the mechanisms previously described resulting in the production of positive and negative ions. On the average, about 34 electron volts of energy are required to produce an ion pair in the gas. The negative ions (free electrons) immediately migrate toward the positive electrode and the positive ions (ionized atoms of the gas) toward the negative electrode. Since the negative ions are much lighter than the positive ions, they travel at a higher velocity and reach the positive electrode more quickly. This results in a flow of current through the circuit that is measured by the current meter. Since the number of ion pairs produced in the gas is determined by the amount of energy given up by the radiation, the deflection of the current meter is a direct measure of the amount of energy deposited in the gas.

The semiconductor detector may be thought of as a solid state ionization detector. There are several advantages to the use of solid detectors. First of all, solids are much more dense than gases and thus much smaller thicknesses are required to totally absorb incident photons. A second advantage is that in general much less energy is required to produce an ion pair in a solid than a gas. This results in more ion pairs produced by each photon interaction and thus a larger electrical signal providing a more statistically accurate measure of the energy of the photon. Obviously,

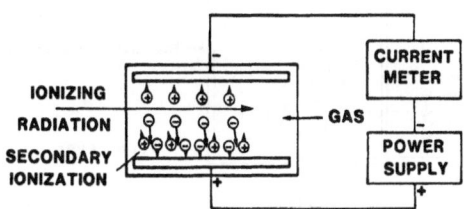

FIGURE 1. Block diagram of a gas-type ionization detector.

34

these advantages also apply to solid scintillation detectors.
However, the use of the scintillation crystal/photomultiplier
tube combination results in statistical fluctuations in the
multiple steps of the detection process which produce
degredations in energy resolution.    These effects are
significantly reduced by the use of semiconductor detector
technology (1).

A schematic of a typical semiconductor detector is shown
in Figure 2.  A semiconductor is defined as a material that
is a very poor conductor of electrical charge.   For each
semiconductor material there exists a critical temperature
below which there are virtually no free charge carriers
present so that the material behaves as an insulator (i.e.,
the material will not conduct an electrical current when a
voltage is applied).   For the two most commonly used
semiconductor materials, silicon (Si) and germanium (Ge),
these critical temperatures are provided by cooling the
materials to the temperature of liquid nitrogen (77° K).
Although the semiconductor materials behave as insulators at
these temperatures, only a very small average amount of
energy (3.72 electron volts for silicon and 2.95 electron
volts for germanium) is required to create an ion pair and
cause a momentary flow of current.

Thus when a photon interaction occurs in a semiconductor
detector, a large number of ion pairs are produced.   These

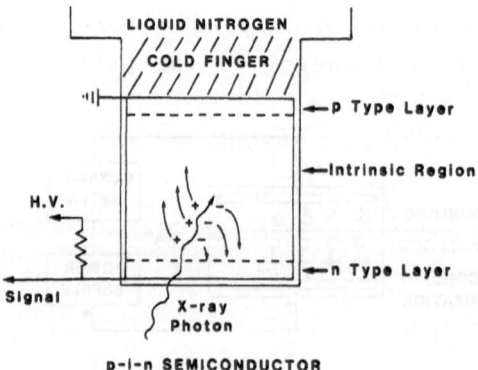

FIGURE 2. Conceptual diagram of a p-i-n semiconductor detector.

are quickly cleared out of the detector by an applied voltage and the collected charge gives rise to an analog voltage pulse whose height is proportional to the energy deposited in the detector by the photon (analogous to the ionization chamber). It is extremely important that all of the free charge produced by the photon interaction be cleared from the detector and collected by the signal electronics. Impurities or imperfections in the detector materials may result in the presence of electrical traps where free charges produced by an interaction can be momentarily or permanently bound and thus alter the magnitude of the signal being produced. It is also imperative that no free charge carriers exist in the detector except in the presence of radiation because this would also alter the detector signal.

It is impossible to manufacture pure silicon crystals to meet the criteria listed above. It is possible, however, to manufacture crystals of silicon which are of the p-type. This means that the material contains an excess of positive charge carriers or "holes". These atoms can then be neutralized by drifting lithium donor atoms (atoms which have an excess of electrons) into the crystal under an applied electric field in order to perfectly compensate the positive charges. This results in an intrinsic crystal containing virtually no free charge carriers. Detectors of this type are operated at an applied voltage of several hundred volts. In order to prevent charges from the electrical contacts being injected into the crystal, it is necessary to coat opposite faces of the detector with p-type (excess "holes") and n-type (excess of electrons) impurities. This process forms a p-i-n junction, in which the i refers to the sensitive volume or intrinsic region and p and n refer to the contacts. The application of a high voltage across the detector then draws out any charge carriers from the region resulting in the creation of a strong electric field across the sensitive intrinsic region.

Lithium atoms are highly mobile at room temperature. Thus lithium-drifted silicon (Si[Li]) detectors tend to undrift and deteriorate when allowed to warm up for extended periods of time. However, current manufacturing techniques now permit multiple short term temperature cyclings with little or no apparent damage.

In years past, lithium-drifted germanium has also been produced by the techniques described above. However, it is now possible to produce crystals of intrinsic germanium in which the impurity levels have been reduced to the point where the compensation process is no longer necessary. The primary advantage of intrinsic germanium for the user is the fact that liquid nitrogen temperatures must be maintained only when the detector is in operation. Temperature cycling will not harm the detector.

A cross-section of a typical semiconductor detector system is shown in Figure 3. The detector is enclosed in an aluminum can with an ultra-thin entrance window. The entrance window is generally made of beryllium, is extremely delicate, and may rupture on contact. The entrance window must be carefully protected because a ruptured window can possibly destroy the detector. The area surrounding the detector is a vacuum in order to maintain an ultra-clean environment free of contaminants which would degrade detector

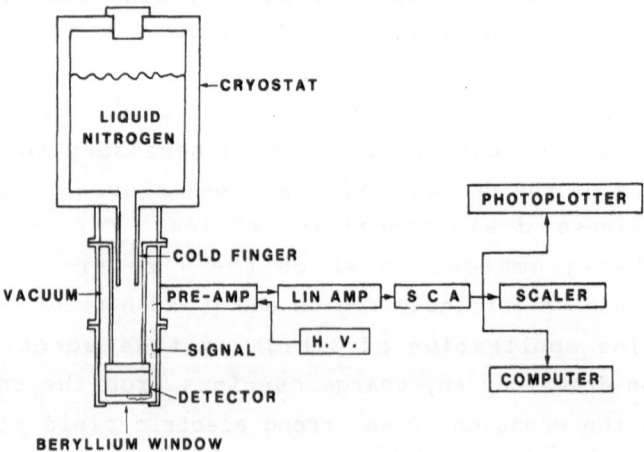

FIGURE 3. Semiconductor detector configuration with signal-processing electronics.

performance. The vacuum is also necessary to maintain the detector at liquid nitrogen temperatures. The detector is coupled directly to a "cold finger" which thermally interfaces the detector to the liquid nitrogen supply. The vacuum is created at the time of manufacture and is maintained by an ion pump or molecular sieve.

For patient applications, the detector is mounted in a vertical configuration using a gravity-fed liquid nitrogen cryostat which is located above the detector. These cryostats are usually of sufficient volume to maintain a 3-4 day supply of liquid nitrogen.

Amplification of signals from the detector is a two stage process. The first stage is accomplished by a pre-amplifier that is located in close proximity to the detector. Since the signals from the detector are extremely low level and relatively noise free, it is imperative that the pre-amplifier be characterized by low noise and high gain. This is usually accomplished through the use of a charge-sensitive pre-amplifier with a field-effect-transistor (FET) as the first component. The FET exhibits extremely low noise characteristics when operated at about 140° K and is therefore often positioned near the detector within the detector enclosure.

The second stage of the amplification process is accomplished by a pulse amplifier. This amplifier must be linear and possess low noise characteristics. It must also be stable and able to handle integral count rates in the range of 20,000-30,000 counts per second. Analog voltage pulses from semiconductor pre-amplifiers are generally in the millivolt range whereas outputs from the pulse amplifier are on the order of 1-5 volts.

After amplification the signals are processed by a single channel analyzer whose purpose is to select only those pulses corresponding to the interactions of the x-ray photons which we wish to count. This instrument must be capable of window selection of 1-2 KeV in width for x-ray fluorescence applications. It must be extremely stable and, along with the pulse amplifier, must be capable of handling a wide range of count rates with no shift in photopeak position. Count rates through the window of a single channel analyzer are typically 100-200 counts per second from a fluorescent system positioned over the thyroid gland in a patient, although the instrument may actually be accepting an integral count rate in excess of 20,000 counts per second. For this reason, considerable attention must be devoted to stability.

The output of the single channel analyzer is a digital pulse or count of 5-10 volts in magnitude and indicates the acceptance of an x-ray photon of the appropriate energy. These digital pulses may be passed to a ratemeter to indicate count rate, to a scaler/timer to measure total counts, to the photoplotter on a rectilinear scanner to produce pictures, or to a computer to record digital information.

Semiconductor detectors are the detectors of choice for x-ray fluorescence applications primarily due to their superior energy resolution. The energy resolution of a semiconductor is typically at least a factor of ten better than that of NaI(Tl) detectors. This is due to the relatively small amount of energy ($\sim 3$ eV) required to produce an ion pair in the semiconductor and also due to the direct collection of charge as a measure of photon energy. In the scintillation detection process, photon energy is converted to light which is then converted to electron flow. The electron flow is then amplified before the final charge collection is performed. Statistical errors in each of these steps lead to degredation in energy resolution. A superior NaI(Tl) scintillation detector will have an energy resolution of 8-9% at 140 KeV whereas a good semiconductor detector will typically have a resolution of less than 1% at that energy. In the x-ray energy range the comparisons are even more dramatic.

A comparison of energy spectra obtained from an I-125 source is shown in Figure 4. The $K_\alpha$ x-ray peak at 27.4 KeV, the $K_\beta$ peak at 31 KeV and the gamma ray peak at 35 KeV are

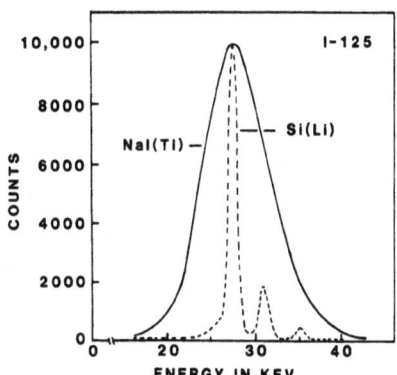

FIGURE 4. Energy spectra obtained with a NaI(Tl) detector and a Si(Li) detector from an I-125 source.

clearly resolved by the Si(Li) detector whereas the NaI(Tl) detector demonstrates only a single peak.

Disadvantages of semiconductors are primarily size and cost related. For x-ray fluorescence applications in patients, detectors have been limited in size to 25 mm diameter by 5 mm thick Si(Li) detectors and 25 mm diameter by 10 mm thick intrinsic germanium detectors. These detectors typically cost $8000-$12,000 with this price including the detector, cryostat, and pre-amplifier.

A problem that has been observed with cryogenically cooled semiconductor systems is microphonics. Under certain circumstances the system may behave as a microphone and respond to loud noises or vibrations by injecting pulses into the counting electronics. These unwanted pulses are electronic noise and therefore degrade energy resolution. This could potentially be a severe problem in moving systems mounted on rectilinear scanners. Careful attention to details in the fabrication process generally eliminates this problem. If microphonic effects are present, they will generally appear in the low energy range. A simple evaluation to perform would be to suspend a low energy source such as I-125 beneath the detector and collect energy spectra with the detector stationary and moving. If no difference is

Table 1. Detector characteristics.

| Detector | Atomic No. | Density (gm/cm$^3$) | Efficiency | | |
|---|---|---|---|---|---|
| | | | 28 KeV | 48 KeV | 140 KeV |
| NaI(T1) (1/2 in) | 50 | 3.67 | 100% | 100% | 100% |
| Si(Li) (5 mm) | 14 | 2.4 | 60% | 20% | 2% |
| HPGe (10 mm) | 32 | 5.4 | 100% | 100% | 75% |

observed when overlaying the spectra, microphonic effects probably are minimal.

For iodine x-ray fluorescence counting and imaging applications involving the thyroid, Si(Li) detectors have generally been the devices of choice. This was partially due to the fact that intrinsic or high purity germanium (HPGe) low energy detectors were not readily available at the time that fluoresence patient studies were initiated. A second reason is that Si(Li) detectors are optimal for low energy work due to their photopeak counting efficiency. Because of the relatively low atomic number and density of silicon (see Table 1), the efficiency of a 5 mm thick Si(Li) detector is 100% up to 16 KeV and then falls off dramatically with increasing energy as shown in Figure 5. It is 60% efficient

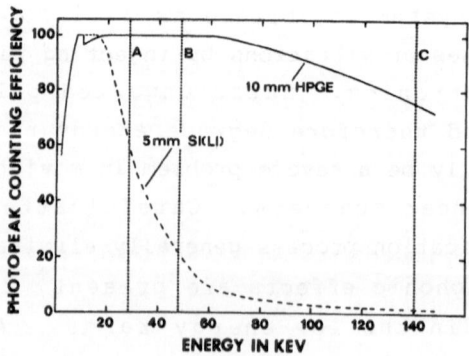

FIGURE 5. Photopeak counting efficiency versus energy for three semiconductor detectors.

at iodine x-ray energies (28.5 KeV) and 20% efficient at 48 KeV (180° Compton-scattered photons from Am-241). Since Compton scatter is the primary source of photons entering the detector (Figure 6), the fewer scatter photons that are absorbed and counted the better. In other words, since less time is spent counting the higher energy Compton-scattered photons, more time can be spent counting the lower energy iodine x-rays.

The source and detector configuration used for fluorescent thyroid imaging at Vanderbilt is shown in Figure 7A. The source consists of 16 individual disk sources, each containing 1 Ci of Am-241, arranged in a circle and individually collimated. The detector is a Si(Li) detector (25 mm diameter, 5 mm thick), manufactured by Ortec, Inc., Oak Ridge, Tennessee. The detector field-of-view is collimated by a single hole tapered to the focal point of the field of irradiation. With this configuration positioned over the thyroid in a patient with a normal iodine distribution, an integral count rate of 20,000 counts per second is obtained (see Table 2). The total count rate through a 1.5 KeV window positioned symmetrically over the iodine x-ray peak with a pulse height analyzer is 200 counts per second. When the system is moved from the thyroid but

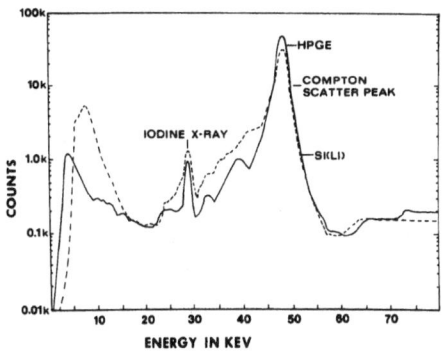

FIGURE 6. Fluorescent energy spectra from a normal thyroidal iodine distribution obtained with a Si(Li) detector and an HPGe detector.

42

Table 2. Detector data from patient measurements.

| Detector | *Energy Resolution | Colli- mator | CPS Integral | CPS Iodine | Window CPS Bkgd | Iodine Bkgd |
|---|---|---|---|---|---|---|
| Si(Li) | 883 KeV | Tapered | 20,000 | 200 | 50 | 4.0 |
| HPGe | ** | Tapered | 65,000 | ** | ** | ** |
| HPGe | 744 KeV | Focused | 20,000 | 100 | 30 | 3.3 |

*Measured FWHM at 27.5 KeV and 1,000 CPS.
**Measurements not given due to severe degredation in resolution
  at this count rate.

still positioned over the neck, a background of 50 counts per
second is obtained due to multiple Compton scatter. This
yields an iodine to background ratio of 4.0. These values
are acceptable for obtaining good quality images of the
thyroid in about 15 minutes of imaging time.

It has been suggested that germanium may provide an
alternative to Si(Li) for x-ray fluorescence scanning of the
thyroid (2). If feasible, this replacement could also permit
the detector system to be used for routine emission scanning
of the thyroid with [$^{99m}$Tc] pertechnetate, due to the
significantly greater efficiency of germanium. This concept

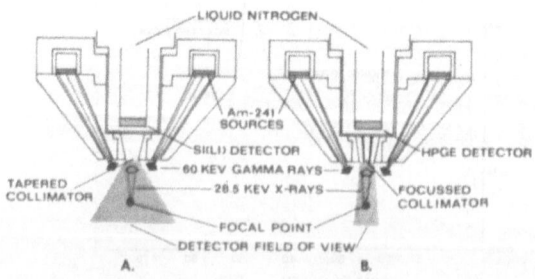

Figure 7. A) Fluorescent source and detector configuration
used for routine patient studies at Vanderbilt Medical Center.
B) Modified configuration for HPGe evaluation.

was evaluated using a 25 mm diameter, 10 mm thick high purity germanium detector in the configuration shown in Figure 7B. Since the integral count rate was excessive (65,000 counts per second), it was necessary to limit the field-of-view of the detector by the use of a multi-hole focused collimator. With this new configuration, the fluorescence spectrum was comparable to that obtained with the Si(Li) detector as shown in Figure 6. Patient measurements yielded an integral count rate of 20,000 counts per second and window count rates of 100 counts per second and 30 counts per second over the thyroid and off the thyroid respectively, for an iodine-to-background ratio of 3.3 (Table 2). These figures were not as good as those for Si(Li); however, acceptable images of the thyroid can be obtained using the germanium detector configuration as shown in Figure 8.

The efficiency of the germanium detector used in this evaluation was 75% at 140 KeV, the primary energy of gamma rays from $^{99m}$Tc. Thus the detector appeared suitable for imaging the pertechnetate distribution in the thyroid as shown by the energy spectrum in Figure 9. Fluorescent and radionuclide images were obtained simultaneously from 5 patients using the HPGe detector and are shown in Figure 10. These images were obtained by using two pulse height analyzers, one processing the iodine x-ray events and the other processing the $^{99m}$Tc gamma ray events, coupled

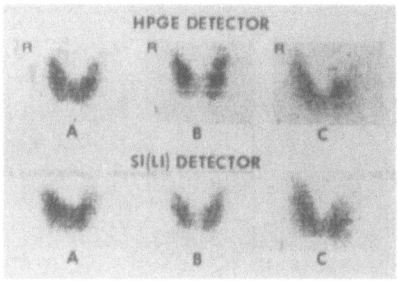

FIGURE 8. XRF scans of three normal volunteers using the two detector configurations shown in FIGURE 7. Identical scanning parameters were used for all studies.

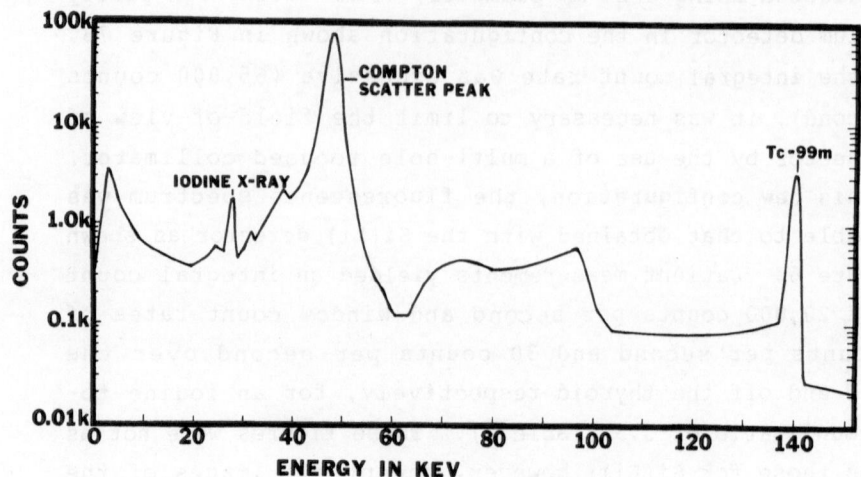

FIGURE 9.. Energy spectrum obtained with the HPGe detector
configuration shown in FIGURE 7B from a source distribution
established to simulate the normal iodine content and uptake
of Tc-99m pertechnetate in the thyroid.

to two separate photoplotters on the rectilinear scanner
imaging system. With the technique, the resolution of the
fluorescent scan is superior due to the double collimation of
both the sources and the detector. However, the resolution
of the radionuclide scan is suffcient to make comparisons
between images. These comparisons should be especially
useful in studies where the stable iodine and radionuclide
distribution differ as in Figures 10D and 10E.

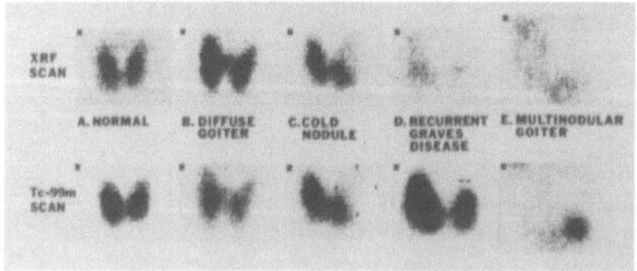

FIGURE 10. Simultaneous XRF and radionuclide scans in five
patients.

Thus it is possible to obtain high quality images of the stable iodine distribution within the thyroid gland using x-ray fluorescent techniques. The lithium-drifted silicon detector is probably the instrument of choice for these applications, although adequate images can be obtained using high purity or intrinsic germanium. Some investigators have reported problems with the latter device (3). However, careful attention to details in the manufacturing process can eliminate these problems (4).

REFERENCES
1. Goulding F, Stone Y. 1971. Semiconductor radiation detectors in Semiconductor Detectors in the Future of Nuclear Medicine. New York, Society of Nuclear Medicine, Inc., pp. 1-15.
2. Patton JA, Brill AB. 1978. Simultaneous emission and fluorescent scanning of the thyroid. J Nucl Med, Vol. 19, pp. 464-469.
3. Palmer DW, Kaufman L, Deconinck F. 1979. Current developments in instrumentation for fluorescent scanning of the thyroid in Medical Applications of Fluorescent Excitation Analysis. Boca Raton, Florida, CRC Press, pp. 139-148.
4. Personal Communication, Ortec, Inc., Oak Ridge, Tennessee, 1979.

IV|A STATIONARY X-RAY FLUORESCENT SYSTEM FOR MEASURING
THYROID IODINE CONCENTRATIONS
S.C. Ng TANG FUI and M.N. MAISEY

In this chapter, we describe a relatively simple X-ray fluorescent system which
we have developed for in-vitro and in-vivo measurement of stable iodine ($^{127}$I) content
in thyroid tissues. The main components of the system are first described followed
by its application for in-vitro and in-vivo investigation. The results of clinical
investigation are finally presented and discussed.

The principle of X-ray fluorescence (XRF) has been described in the first
chapter of the monograph. In brief, if a beam of gamma rays of appropriate
energy is directed towards an iodine containing target such as an iodide solution
or thyroid tissue, the iodine atoms are excited and release characteristic
fluorescent X-ray photons which can be used to identify and measure the
concentration of the element. The energy spectrum emitted from the target
(Fig. l) shows narrow peaks ($K_\alpha$ and $K_\beta$) corresponding to the fluorescent iodine
X-rays and a wider peak resulting from Comptom scattering of the incident
gamma rays. The counts in the $K_\alpha$ peak are proportional to the iodine content of
the target.

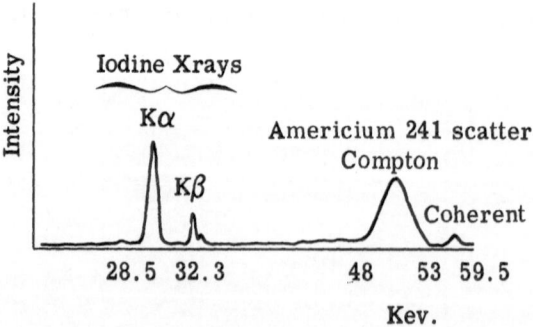

Fig. l Energy spectrum of photons emitted during irradiation of iodine target

INSTRUMENTATION

The basic components of an XRF system thus consist of (a) an external source of exciting gamma rays, (b) a detector of high resolution capable of detecting and separating the low energy fluorescent X-rays, (c) an amplifier and (d) an analyser to identify and quantitate the iodine X-rays.

Figs. 2(a) and (b) illustrate the various components of our stationary system and the set-up for in-vitro and in-vivo investigation respectively.

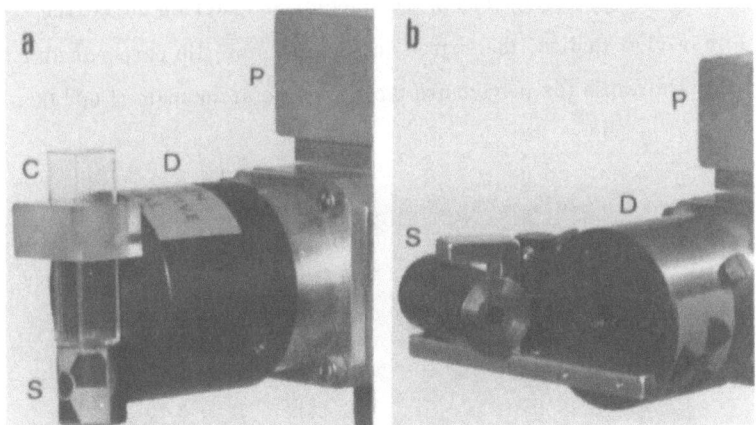

Fig. 2   Main components of stationary XRF system  (a) for in-vitro use (b) for in-vivo use.   S = source    D = detector    P = pre-amplifier C = cuvette for sample

(a)  The source

A sealed source of 300 mCi (11 GBq) of Americium 241 ($^{241}$Am) supplied by the Radiochemical Centre, Amersham, England, is used to provide a beam of 59.5 Kev gamma rays. The source is enclosed in a discoid steel capsule, one surface of which serves as a 0.2 mm thick window through which the exciting beam emerges towards the target. For in-vitro investigations, the encapsulated source is placed in a shallow cylindrical lead container (Fig. 2a) which serves as a straight single hole collimator for the exciting beam. For in-vivo studies the latter is replaced by a converging single hole lead collimator to "focus" the beam towards the centre of one lobe of the thyroid.

(b) The detector

A silicon (Lithium drifted) semi-conductor detector, obtained from Kevex
Corporation, California, USA, is used. It is a 3 mm thick disc with a sensitive
surface area 80 mm$^2$ mounted at the anterior end of a horizontal steel hollow
cylinder (Fig. 3) which is cooled by liquid nitrogen contained in a Dervar drum.
A thin Bery lium window lies immediately in front of the anterior surface of the
detector. A collar type cylindrical steel attachment with a central aperture 8 mm
in diameter fits over the anterior end of the detector and carries the source at
an angle. For in-vivo studies, the source and the detector, lie perpendicular to
each other (Fig. 2a) while for in-vivo use their axes lie at an angle of 60° in a
horizontal plane (Fig. 2b).

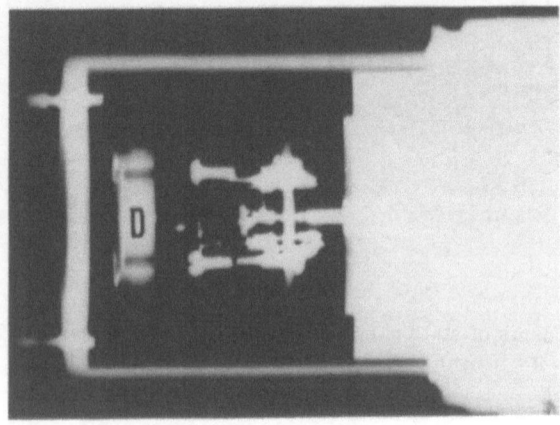

Fig. 3   Radiograph of the anterior end of detector to show the position of the
Si (Li) disc   (D)

(c) Pre-amplifier and amplifier

The electronic signals from the detector are fed to a pre-amplifier (Kevex
Model 2003) situated on top of the cylindrical arm of the detector and then to the
main amplifier (Tennelec Model Tc 205 A). When operational the amplifier is
usually set at a gain of 500.

(d)  Analyser

A 1024 multichannel analyser (Nuclear Data Model ND 100) incorporating an analogue to digital convertor (ND 500) displays the emitted spectrum on an oscilloscope screen.  By adjusting electronic markers the count within the $K_\alpha$ iodine peak can be read on the alphanumeric display on the upper part of the screen.

IN VITRO MEASUREMENT

(a)  Sample preparation

We have used the stationary system to measure the iodine concentration in normal thyroid tissue obtained at post-mortem and pathological specimens excised during surgical operations.  The specimens which were usually fixed in formalin were dried carefully with filter paper, from which three representative portions each about a gram were cut out, weighed individually and incubated at $80^\circ C$ with an equal amount (w/v) of molar sodium hydroxide until completely dissolved (Tadros, 1978).  This resulted in extracts containing a two-fold dilution of the intrathyroidal iodine concentration.  One ml of each extract was placed in a disposable plastic cuvette and irradiated on the XRF system for iodine measurement.  A calibration curve was obtained by irradiating one ml samples of serial dilutions of a standard solution of potassium iodide.

(b)  Technique of measurement

Iodine estimation was carried out according to the method of Moss et al (1972). The cuvette containing the sample was positioned in the right angle between the $^{241}$Am source and the anterior surface of the detector (Fig. 2a).  The sample was thus irradiated from below, each for 100 seconds, and the emitted photons detected in a perpendicular direction.  The counts in the $K_\alpha$ peak of iodine were recorded and the background count subtracted from the horizontal segment between the $K_\alpha$ and $K\beta$ peaks.  The mean value of the corrected counts for the three samples from each thyroid specimen was calculated and the corresponding iodine concentration derived from the calibration curve.

(c) <u>Results</u>

Fig. 4 shows the calibration curve for the standard potassium iodide solutions. The counts in the $K_\gamma$ peak show a linear relationship with the iodine concentration in the standard solution. Using a 99% confidence limit, the minimum detectable concentration of iodine in the cuvette was 0.01 mg/ml corresponding to 0.02 mg/ml of thyroid tissue.

Fig. 5 shows the iodine concentration derived by this technique for 46 normal thyroids and 88 pathological specimens with various histological diagnoses. No iodine was detected in the formalin fixing solution, thus excluding any significant leakage of iodine from the thyroid specimens.

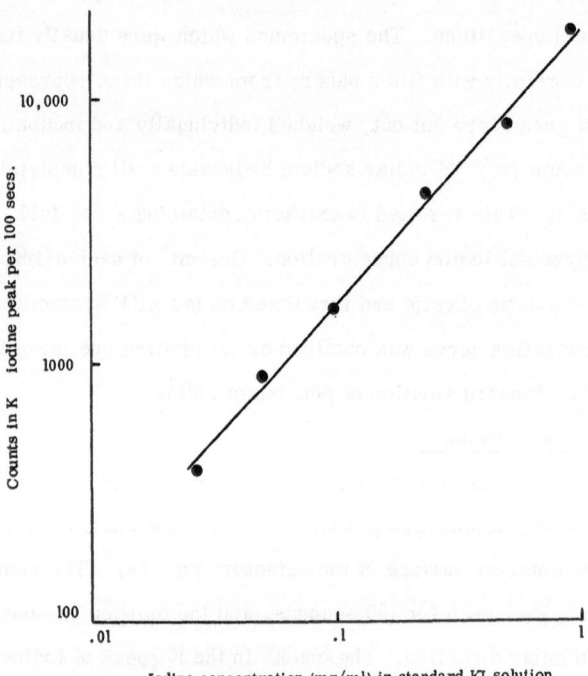

<u>Fig. 4</u>    Calibration curve for standard iodide solution

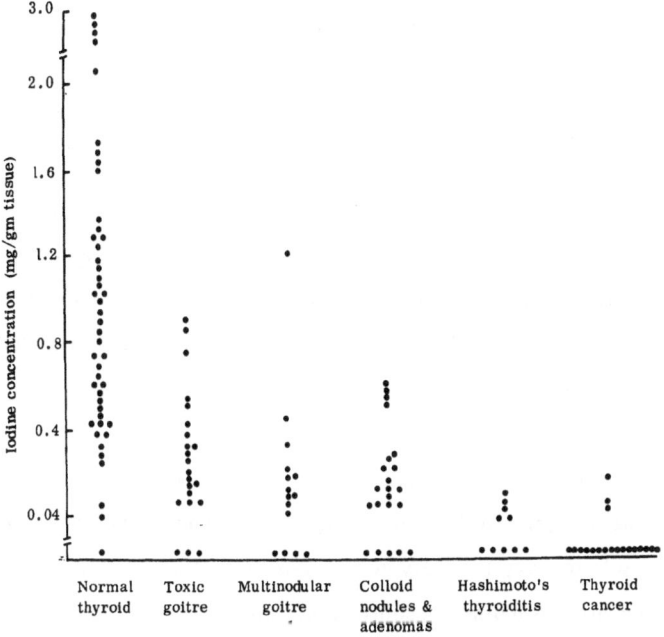

Iodine concentration in normal and pathological thyroid tissues

__Fig. 5__  Iodine concentrations in normal and pathological thyroids.
ND = Not detectable        MNG = Multinodular goitre

(d)  Discussion

Our results indicate a mean iodine concentration of 1.03 $\pm$ 0.67 mg/gm of tissue (range 0.02 to 3.12 mg/gm) in normal thyroids.  This is not significantly different from the mean normal level of 0.98 mg/gm reported by Le Blanc et al (1973) in Texas using an in-vitro XRF technique or that found by Fisher and Oddie (1969) using chemical methods (1.03 mg/gm).  Comparable values were observed from in-vivo radioiodine clearance studies by the same investigators.  Statistical analysis of our data showed no significant variation with age (25 to 80 years) or sex.  Our results like those of Le Blanc et al (1973) and Fisher and Oddie (1969) show that there is considerable individual variation in normal thyroids, the cause of which is unknown.

The mean iodine concentration for each pathological tissue type was significantly lower than the mean normal value but there was some degree of overlap between the ranges of values for each histological group. Thus iodine concentration was not significantly different in toxig goitres, multinodular goitres and solitary benign nodules. This contrasts with the difference in radioiodine uptake usually seen in these conditions, high in diffuse toxic goitre and low in benign non-functioning nodules, indicating that iodine storage in the thyroid is not directly related to its iodine uptake as previously noted by Thrall et al (1977). There is thus no diagnostic relationship between iodine concentration and any of these three types of thyroid disease. In Hashimoto's thyroiditis however, the iodine concentration is consistently low as previously noted by Hoffer et al (1971) and may therefore be of diagnostic value.

The lowest iodine concentration in the present study was found in thyroid cancer. 16 (84%) of the 19 malignant nodules examined had undetectable iodine stores (less than 0.02 mg/gm); in the remaining 3 specimens iodine concentration was only just detectable or very low. By comparison 96% of the benign nodules we examined had measurable iodine concentration, ranging from 0.02 to 0.68 mg/gm of tissue indicating that benign nodules are able to store iodine more efficiently than the malignant tumours, though less efficiently than normal thyroid tissue.

In vitro studies by Le Blanc et al (1973) also showed that the mean iodine concentration was lower in malignant (0.12 mg/gm) than in benign nodules (0.20 mg/gm). However the range of values for their benign and malignant nodules showed a greater degree of overlap than in our study. 55% (6 out of 11) of their thyroid cancer specimens had undetectable iodine stores compared to only 21% (3 out of 14) of the benign nodules. However it should be pointed out that they used a proportional counter to detect the emitted photons and the sensitivity of their system was less than ours; their lowest detectable iodine concentration was 0.04 mg/gm compared to 0.02 mg/gm for our system.

Our in-vitro findings suggest that measurement of iodine content of solitary nodules in-vivo may be of value in differentiating between benign and malignant lesions pre-operatively. The absence of any detectable iodine stores would increase the probability of malignancy whereas the finding of significant amount of iodine would reduce its risk. This is further discussed in the next section.

## IN-VIVO STUDIES

### Adaptation and validation of technique

Following the encouraging results obtained with our in-vitro studies, we have extended the use of the stationary XRF system to in-vivo measurement of iodine content of regional areas of the thyroid such as a palpable nodule or a localised area of a diffuse goitre. Some modification of the system was found necessary and Figs. 6 - 10 illustrate the work-up during the adaptation and validation of the technique for in-vivo use.

A model of the neck and thyroid gland (Fig. 6) was constructed as follows.

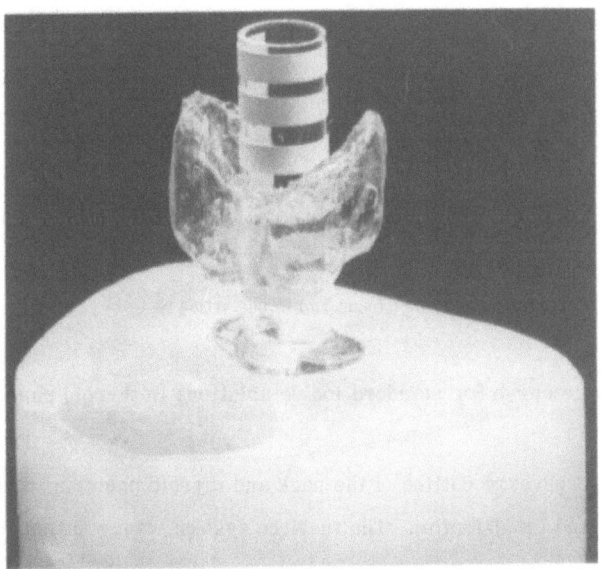

Fig. 6   Phantom of neck and thyroid

A perspex hollow cast of a normal sized thyroid gland was carefully prepared by Dr. M. Hutchinson of the Anatomy Department, Guy's Hospital Medical School, who has considerable expertise in this field. The two lobes of the thyroid cast were partitioned by a midline septum so that potassium iodide solutions of varying concentrations could be filled into each lobe independently through a hole in the upper edge. A wax phantom of an average female neck was provided by our Radiotherapy Department where such phantoms are routinely prepared for patients

undergoing radiotherapy for head and neck tumours. The neck phantom contains
a cavity anteriorly into which the thyroid cast could be inserted.

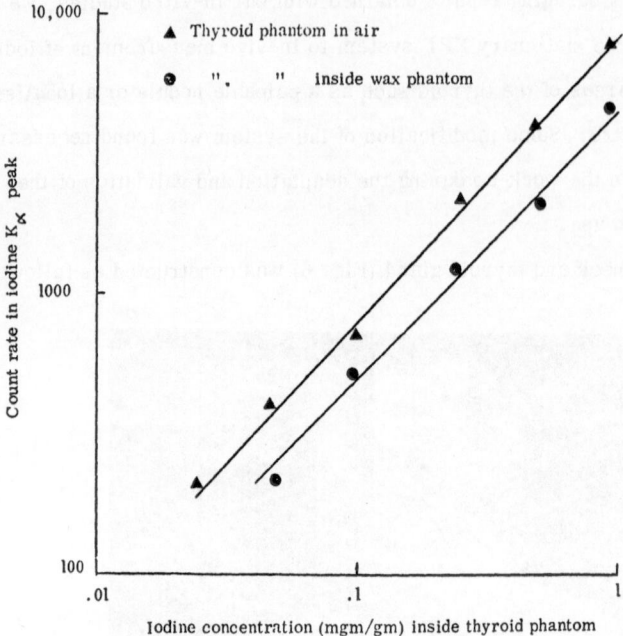

**Fig. 7**   Dose response curve for standard iodide solutions in thyroid phantom

Fig. 8 shows a transverse outline of the neck and thyroid phantom in relation
to the $^{241}$Am source and the detector. The in-vitro system was modified in two
ways for in-vivo investigation. First the angle between the source and the detector
(which was 90° for in-vitro study) was made more acute so that they could both
point towards one lobe of the thyroid. An angle of 60° was found to be most
suitable for the average female neck, but this angle can be adjusted according to
the size and shape of individual patients' necks. Secondly, the cylindrical
collimator for the source used in in-vitro studies was replaced by a converging
single hole collimator so that the exciting beam could be "focused" to a point
approximately in the centre of one lobe of the thyroid model. The neck is
positioned so that one lobe of the gland lies in the angle between the source and
the detector, as shown in Fig. 8. To investigate the opposite lobe the source is
rotated through 180° in a vertical plane by means of the collar attachment around

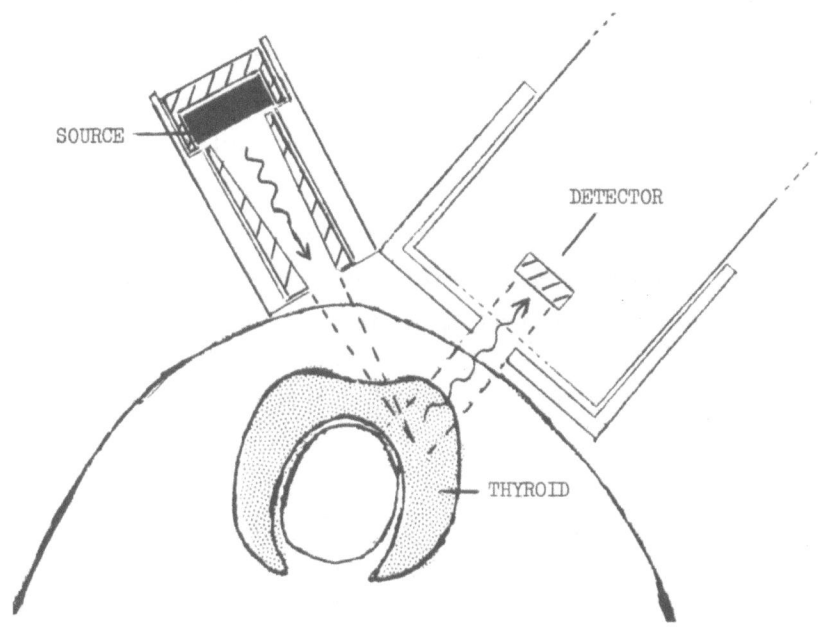

Fig. 8  Transverse outline of neck and thyroid phantom with source and detector.

the detector and the neck is re-positioned to maintain the same geometrical
relationship between the source, the detector and the opposite lobe.

The following experiments were carried out to validate the in-vivo technique:

Experiment 1

One lobe of the thyroid phantom was filled with a standard potassium iodide
solution. The opposite lobe was initially kept empty. The count rate in the iodine
$K_\alpha$ peak obtained by irradiating the filled-in lobe was recorded for varying
standard potassium iodide concentrations ranging from 0.01 to 10 mg/ml. Fig. 7
shows the dose-response curve with the thyroid phantom in air and then in the
neck phantom. A linear relationship was maintained but as expected the count
rate is reduced with the thyroid in the neck phantom due to absorption of the
incident and emitted photons by the overlying thickness of wax. Addition of
potassium iodide solution in the opposite lobe made no significant difference to
the dose response curve for the left lobe.

## Experiment 2

In order to assess the regional size of the thyroid examined by our system, defined by the intersention of the exciting beam and the field of view of the detector (Hoffer et al, 1971; Tinney 1971), an isocount plot was carried out as follows. A thin plastic catheter 15 cms long mounted vertically was filled with a strong iodide solution and placed at various positions in the "field of view" of the system. The count rate per 100 seconds was measured in each position and an isocount plot was obtained, as shown in Fig. 9. Counting was repeated with the iodide line

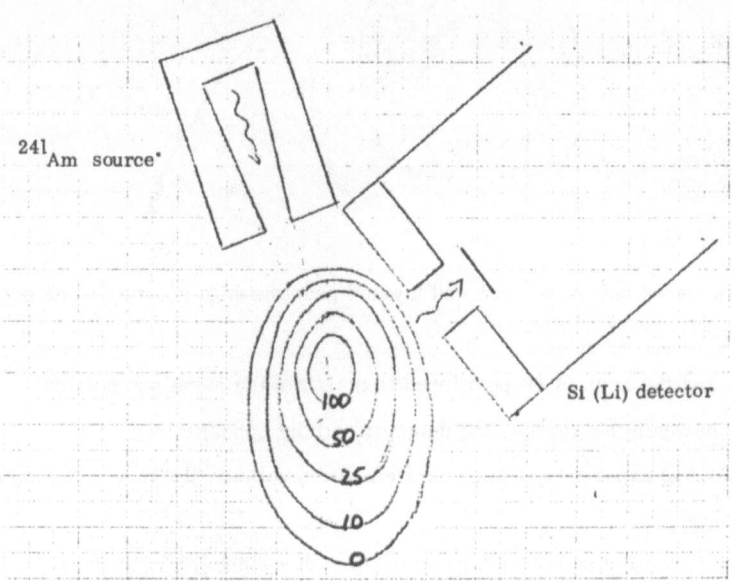

$^{241}$Am source

Si (Li) detector

**Fig. 9** Isocount plot with line target in air

target immersed in a plastic cylindrical container, 5 inches in diameter, filled with water. Fig. 10 shows the isocount plot in water. These experiments suggest that the system has a sensitive field of view of about 2.5 to 3 cms in diameter.

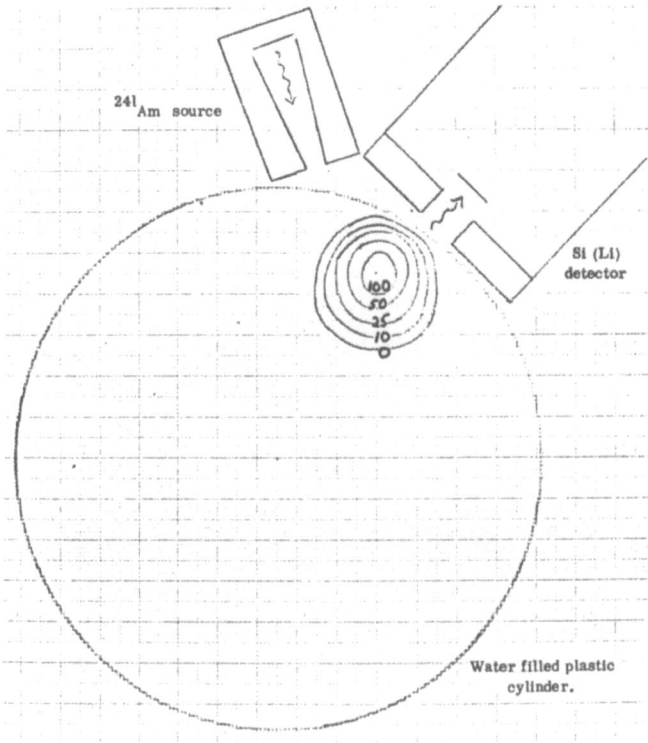

**Fig. 10** Isocount plot with line target in water cylinder

### Clinical Investigation

The in-vivo technique has been used to investigate patients with normal and pathological thyroids referred to the Nuclear Medicine Department for routine radionuclide scanning. The study was approved by the Guy's Hospital Medical School Ethical Committee and informed consent was obtained from each patient prior to the fluorescent examination. In each case, iodine measurement was carried out before any radionuclide was administered to the patient for the routine scan.

The procedure was fully explained to each patient. The neck was first carefully palpated to define the position and size of the thyroid and any palpable nodule was marked. The source and detector were carefully positioned so that they both pointed towards the lobe under investigation and away from the opposite lobe.

58

When the thyroid was not palpable, the position was adjusted until the maximum count rate was observed on the rate meter of the analyser. Inaccuracies can result from inadequate positioning.

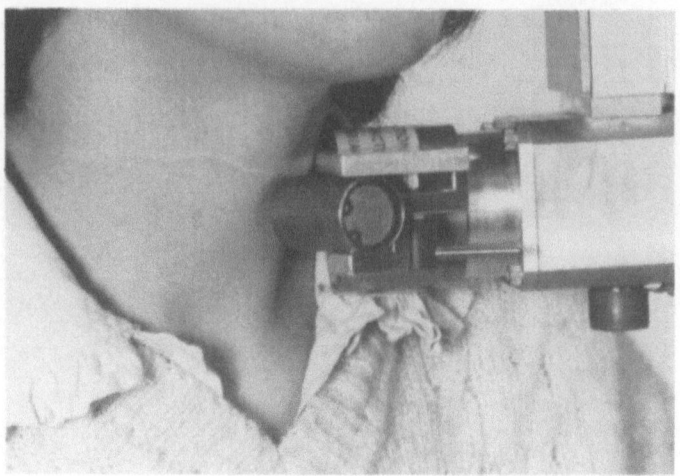

Fig. 11  The system in-position to investigate the left lobe

Fig. 11 shows the position of the patient with respect to the source and detector when investigating the left lobe. To investigate the opposite lobe, the patient rotates through $180^{\circ}$ horizontally while the attachment of the source and detector is rotated through $180^{\circ}$ in a vertical plane. Counting was carried out for 100 seconds on each side. Fig. 12 shows the $K_{\alpha}$ iodine peak from a patient with a normal thyroid.

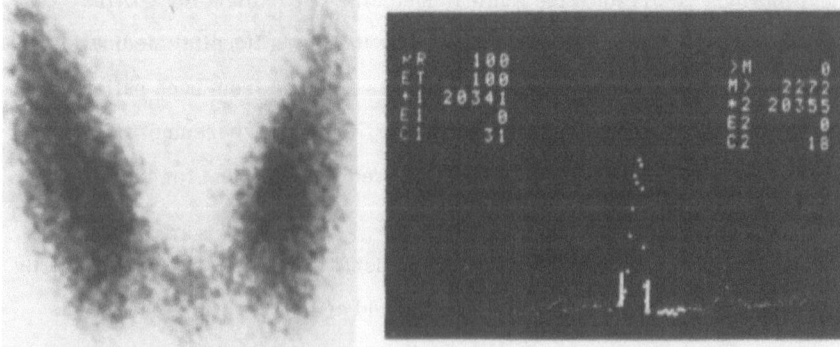

Fig. 12  (a) Normal $^{99}Tc^m$ thyroid scan.  (b) $K_{\alpha}$ iodine peak from same patient during XRF study.

The iodine content is expressed as count rate per 100 seconds in the $K_\alpha$ peak instead of absolute units of concentration due to the difficulty with in-vivo calibration and the variability of the conversion factor for individual patients caused by such variables as skin thickness, size and shape of the thyroid. The results for individual patients are not therefore strictly comparable, and the findings may only be considered an approximate guide to the true iodine content in the thyroid tissues.

Over 200 patients have been studied by the in-vivo technique, but for the purpose of this report only those whose diagnosis has been confirmed surgically or otherwise will be reported. These include (1) normal thyroids, (2) thyroglossal cysts, (3) thyroid cancer, (4) benign solitary cold nodules, (5) functioning nodules, (6) diffuse toxic goitre, (7) flooded iodine pool.

## RESULTS

### Normal thyroid

20 patients considered to have normal thyroids were examined. All were clinically and biochemically euthyroid and had no thyroid abnormality on palpation or on $^{99}Tc^m$ scan. These patients were referred to the Nuclear Medicine Department either for a salivary gland scan with $^{99}Tc^m$ so that the thyroid could be imaged simultaneously or for a $^{99}Tc^m$ thyroid scan to exclude a thyroid abnormality for various symptoms in the neck. Fig. 13 shows the count rate in the $K_\alpha$ iodine peak for each lobe of the thyroid from these 20 patients. Iodine was detectable in all cases though there was considerable variation as previously noted in our in-vitro studies. For any particular patient the count rate was approximately equal for the two lobes of the thyroid.

### Thyroglossal cysts

Three children with thyroglossal cysts, confirmed surgically, were studied pre-operatively. The fluorescent examination showed no stable iodine in the cyst but confirmed the presence of a normal thyroid in the usual position in the neck by its stable iodine content.

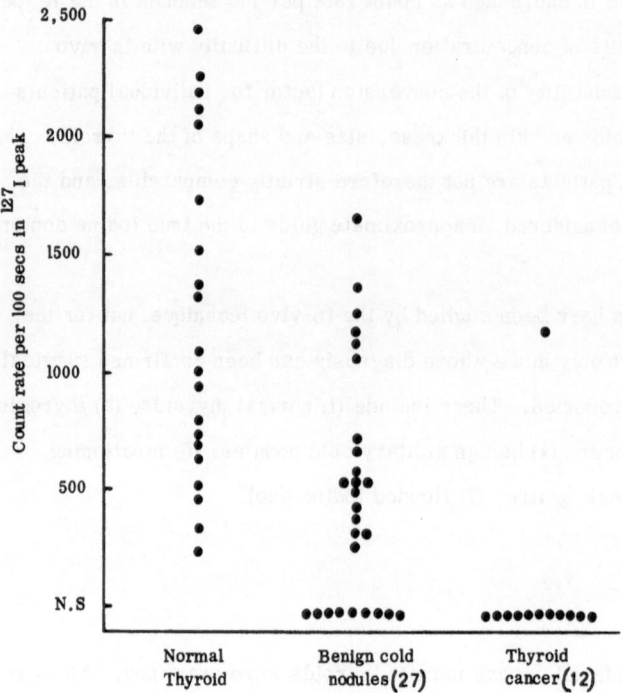

<u>Fig. 13</u>  Iodine content in thyroids measured by in-vivo XRF technique

### Thyroid cancer

12 patients with histologically proven thyroid cancer (11 differentiated and
one anaplastic tumour) were studied by the in-vivo XRF system.  9 of these patients
were new cases who presented with a solitary thyroid nodule greater than 2.5 cms
in diameter, shown to be cold on $^{99}Tc^m$ scan.  The fluorescent study showed
undetectable iodine in all but one of the nodules.  The opposite normal lobes all
had normal iodine counts.  3 patients were studied when they presented with
recurrent tumour in the neck after previous surgical and radioiodine ablation.
Stable iodine was undetectable in all 3 recurrent malignant nodules although the
whole body radioiodine scan showed significant radioiodine uptake in the nodule.

### Benign solitary cold nodules  (Table I)

27 patients with benign solitary cold nodules >2.5 cm in diameter were studied
pre-operatively.  Stable iodine was measurable in 18 of these nodules but
undetectable in the remaining 9.  Stable iodine was undetectable in 4 thyroid cysts

in-vivo and on the aspirated fluid from them.

Table I    Count rate per 100 seconds in $K_\alpha$ iodine peak in solitary "hot" nodules and contralateral lobes.

|  | Patient | Nodule | Opp. lobe |
|---|---|---|---|
| (a) Toxic | D.B. | 749 | 805 |
|  | A.B. | N.S. | N.S. |
|  | M.D. | 463 | 475 |
|  | G.E. | 1029 | N.S. |
|  | H.R. | 441 | N.S. |
|  | L.T. | 1022 | 469 |
|  | N.W. | 288 | N.S. |
| (b) Non-toxic | D.C. | 419 | 230 |
|  | R.E. | 592 | N.S. |
|  | L.S. | 1377 | 750 |
|  | E.V. | 266 | 594 |

N.S. = Not significant

### Hot nodules

11 patients with solitary autonomously functioning nodules were examined. None was removed surgically. 7 of these patients were also hyperthyroid and in 5 of these the toxic nodule had measurable iodine stores with count rates ranging from 400 to 1000 per 100 seconds. The other 2 toxic nodules had undetectable stable iodine stores despite good radioiodine uptake. On the other hand, the contralateral suppressed lobe had detectable iodine stores in 3 but not in 4 of the toxic patients.

In 4 patients the autonomous nodule was not associated with hyperthyroidism; in all cases stable iodine was detectable in significant quantities. The partially suppressed contralateral lobe contained iodine in 3 of the 4 patients.

### Diffuse toxic goitre

19 patients with newly diagnosed diffuse toxic goitre (Graves' disease) were studied. The results of the iodine content in each lobe for each patient are shown in Table II. 12 patients had count rates ranging from 700 to 2500 in either lobe, representing normal or high iodine stores; 3 patients however had undetectable iodine in either lobe despite high $^{99}Tc^m$ uptake on the radionuclide scan. 4 patients had detectable iodine in only one lobe.

Table II  Count rate per 100 seconds in $K_\alpha$ iodine peak in patients with diffuse
toxic goitre

| Patient | Right lobe | Left lobe |
|---------|-----------|-----------|
| E.A. | 2356 | 2414 |
| S.A. | N.S. | N.S. |
| C.B. | N.S. | N.S. |
| J.B. | 1540 | 768 |
| P.B. | 912 | N.S. |
| S.F. | 893 | 1087 |
| E.F. | 2603 | 2522 |
| D.G. | 815 | 607 |
| H.H. | 933 | 846 |
| A.K. | 235 | 248 |
| A.L. | 1509 | 1979 |
| K.O. | N.S. | 869 |
| S.P. | N.S. | N.S. |
| D.P. | 1052 | 1286 |
| R.R. | 672 | 913 |
| J.R. | 895 | N.S. |
| E.S. | 979 | 1320 |
| E.SA. | 857 | 569 |
| M.T. | 1152 | N.S. |

N.S. = Not significant

## Flooded iodine pool

2 patients with a solitary nodule were found to have complete absence of
$99Tc^m$ uptake on the radionuclide scan because they had received iodinated X-ray
contrast media shortly before they were referred for the thyroid scan. Fluorescent
studies showed no $127I$ in one nodule, subsequently shown to be malignant, but the
other nodule which was benign had detectable iodine stores. Iodine was detectable
in the contralateral normal lobe in both patients despite the absence of any $99Tc^m$
uptake. A repeat $99Tc^m$ scan six weeks later showed normal uptake in the normal
lobe but the nodules were cold and thus excised.

## DISCUSSION

We have shown that a relatively simple stationary XRF system such as the one
we describe can be used to investigate the iodine content in thyroid tissues both in
vitro and in-vivo. Though the same set-up that we use for in-vivo investigation
can also be used for in-vitro measurement, the sensitivity of the system is better
and positioning of the sample in the cuvette is easier with the source and detector

set perpendicular to each other as shown in Fig. 2(a). It should be pointed out that whereas the in-vitro technique provides quantitative estimation of the iodine concentration in the samples measured, the in-vivo method only provides a semi-quantitative assessment of the iodine content in the volume of tissue within the field of view of the source and the detector. This was estimated to have a diameter of approximately 2.5 to 3.0 cms (Ng Tang Fui, 1979). When the system is used to investigate nodules or other parts of the thyroid of 3.0 cms in diameter or more, the iodine count rate approximately reflects iodine concentration but is subject to inaccuracies resulting from variation in skin thickness and any normal thyroid tissue overlying the region under investigation. These features limit the quantitative value of the technique. Compared to a fluorescent scanner, our stationary system has the main disadvantage of not providing an image of the entire thyroid gland or of the part under investigation. Instead it concentrates on a localised area of the thyroid of particular interest such as a palpable nodule or part of a lobe of a diffuse goitre for which it can provide semi-quantitative information on iodine stores.

The stationary system is simpler, cheaper and more compact than the scanner. It does not require as strong a source as the scanner; the study time is short and the radiation dose to the thyroid though quite low with the fluorescent scanner - approximately 15 millirads per scan (Hoffer et al, 1971) - is reduced even further (2 millirads per patient in our study).

The results of our in-vivo studies show several interesting features. Normal thyroids have the considerable variation in iodine content noted in our in-vitro studies and in other studies (Le Blanc et al, 1973; Fisher and Oddie, 1969). The explanation is not clear. None of the patients studied had a fat neck to account for the low values obtained in some.

The investigation of children with thyroglossal cysts shows a definite useful clinical application of the fluorescent technique using either a scanner or a stationary system. These cysts may be confused with ectopic thyroids and misdiagnosis may lead to excision of the patient's only thyroid tissue and result in hypothyroidism. It is thus essential to establish that a normal thyroid is present before excising a suspected thyroglossal cyst. A radionuclide scan is usually advised but a fluorescent study either with a scanner or more simply with a stationary system provides a better alternative (due to the lower radiation dose) by demonstrating the presence of normal iodine stores in the usual position of the thyroid but not in the cyst.

Our results confirm the usefulness of fluorescent thyroid studies in patients who have received large quantities of iodine compounds such as radiological contrast media when conventional radionuclide scan is unable to image the thyroid due to the excess iodine pool. Fluorescent study is still possible under these circumstances since it is not dependent on circulating iodine but on the intra-thyroidal stable iodine content which is not significant disturbed by the excess circulating iodine. Both our patients who had contrast media had measurable levels of stable iodine in the normal lobe which could not be imaged by the $^{99}Tc^m$ scan but imaging would have been successful with a fluorescent scanner.

Fluorescent studies may also be useful in patients with hot (functioning) nodules to investigate the contralateral lobe. In such patients, particularly if the nodule is causing hyperthyroidism, the opposite lobe is often not visualised on the radionuclide scan and it is therefore not possible to distinguish whether the lobe is absent or suppressed except after TSH stimulation (Ng Tang Fui and Maisey, 1979). Fluorescent studies carried out during the initial investigation however can establish the presence of the contralateral lobe by the presence of its stable iodine store. This was possible in 3 of our 4 patients with a toxic nodule. A combination of fluorescent and radionuclide studies during one visit can thus provide full morphological and functional assessment of the thyroid with a toxic nodule. However the toxic nodule itself may contain an increased, decreased or normal stable iodine store and fluorescent study is therefore not useful in diagnosing its hyperfunctioning nature. The limitation of the diagnostic value of the fluorescent scan is also reflected in the assessment of diffuse toxic goitre, since the stable iodine content may be normal, increased or occasionally even decreased as shown by several investigations (Hoffer et al, 1971; Jonckheer and Deconinck, 1979) and confirmed by our findings. However in the presence of hyperthyroidism confirmed biochemically, the fluorescent scan will show the diffuseness of the iodine store in patients with Graves' disease. The possibility that X-ray fluorescent study may be useful in predicting the chances of relapse or remission after anti-thyroid therapy in Graves' disease has also been suggested

(Hoffer et al, 1971).

The results of our in-vivo investigation of benign and malignant thyroid nodules suggest that quantitative measurement of iodine content by XRF may be helpful in the pre-operative differentiation of solitary cold nodules. I-127 was undetectable in 90% (11 out of 12) of the malignant nodules we studied in-vivo compared to only 33% of the benign cold nodules. The majority of the benign nodules (67%) had detectable iodine stores at low or medium ranges of concentration. Comparable results were obtained in our in-vitro studies but the better in-vitro sensitivity enabled low iodine concentration to be detected in a comparatively higher proportion of benign and malignant nodules.

An even higher degree of separation of benign and malignant nodules has been reported by Patton et al (1976) who used an in-vivo computerised fluorescent scanning system to estimate the ratio of I-127 content of solitary cold nodules to that of the opposite normal lobe. They found that a ratio of less than 0.6 distinguished the malignant nodules from the benign ones with an accuracy of 90%. While our stationary system does not differentiate benign and malignant nodules with such a high degree of confidence, the results do support an increased risk of malignancy in nodules with undetectable iodine compared to those with measurable levels. We conclude that solitary thyroid nodules that are cold on radionuclide scan, solid on ultrasound examination and devoid of iodine on XRF study should be excised as they carry the highest risk of malignancy.

## REFERENCES

1. Fisher DA and Oddie TM. 1969. Thyroid iodine content and turnover in euthyroid subjects. Validity of estimation of thyroid iodine accumulation from short tem clearance studies. Journal of Clinical Endocrinology, 29, 721.
2. Hoffer PB, Bernstein J and Gottschalk A. 1971. Fluorescent techniques in thyroid imaging. Seminars in Nuclear Medicine, 1, 379.
3. Hoffer PB, Gottschalk and Foster J. 1971. Fluorescent thyroid scanning. Initial clinical results. Radiology, 99, 117.
4. Jonckheer M and Deconinck F. 1979. Dissociation between iodine storage function and hormone formation as observed with XRF scanning of the thyroid. 10th Annual Meeting of the European Thyroid Association. Annales d'endocrinologie, t,40, 45.
5. Le Blanc AD, Bell RL and Johnson PC. 1973. Measurement of $^{127}$I concentration in thyroid tissue by X-ray fluorescence. Journal of Nuclear Medicine, 14, 816.

66

6.  Moss AA, Kaufman L and Nelson JA. 1972. Fluorescent excitation analysis:
    A simplified method of iodine determination in vitro. Investigative Radiology,
    7, 335.
7.  Ng Tang Fui S. 1979. The in-vivo measurement of stable iodine in the thyroid
    by X-ray fluorescence. MSc thesis, London University.
8.  Ng Tang Fui S and Maisey MN. 1979. Standard dose $^{131}$I therapy for hyper-
    thyroidism caused by autonomously functioning thyroid nodules. Clinical
    Endocrinology, 10, 69.
9.  Patton JA, Hollifield JW, Brill AB, Lee GS and Patton DD. 1976.
    Differentiation between malignant and benign solitary thyroid nodules by
    fluorescent scanning. Journal of Nuclear Medicine, 17, 17.
10. Tadros TG. 1978. Fluorescent excitation analysis in clinical and endo-
    crinological investigations. PhD thesis, University of London.
11. Thrall JM, Burman KD, Gillin MT, Corcoran RJ, Johnson MC and
    Wantofsky L. 1977. Solitary autonomous thyroid nodules : comparison of
    fluorescent and pertechnetate imaging. Journal of Nuclear Medicine, 18, 1064.
12. Tinney JF. 1971. In-vivo X-ray fluorescent analysis - Concepts and equipment.
    In Semiconductor detectors in the future of nuclear medicine. Ed. Hoffer PB,
Beck RN and Gottschalk A. Publ. The Society of Nuclear Medicine Inc, New York.

# V QUANTIFICATION PROBLEMS IN X-RAY FLUORESCENCE DETERMINATION OF INTRATHYROIDAL IODINE

A. MAGRINI, L. RAGANELLA, S. DI LUZIO, G. IZZO, P. PAVONI

## 1. INTRODUCTION

The "in vivo" measurement of total intrathyroidal stable iodine by X-ray fluorescence (XRF) was originally considered as a means of collecting additional information making use of an XRF device (fluorescent scanner) designed primarily for thyroid imaging (1-6).

Later, non-imaging (static) XRF devices were employed for the sole purpose of iodine quantitation (7,8). A device of this type was also used in the dynamic study of thyroid uptake following the administration of stable iodine (9,10).

The main advantage of non-imaging vs imaging XRF devices is the marked reduction in the cost of equipment, since roughly-collimated low-activity ($\leqslant$ 300 mCi) $^{241}$Am source(s) can be employed instead of highly-collimated X-ray tube or high activity (10$\div$20 Ci) $^{241}$Am source(s). The system can be further simplified and costs further reduced by using a proportional gas counter (9) which is much smaller and about ten times less expensive than the most commonly used solid state detectors (Si(Li) and HpGe). Moreover, the former does not need any maintenance while the latter two need to be constantly cooled with liquid nitrogen (Si(Li) needs cooling also when not working).

An analysis of the various XRF devices with respect to their cost and performances in studies on the thyroid (imaging, iodine quantitation and dynamic study) can be found in ref. (10). The present report focuses on the basic physical and technical aspects of intrathyroidal iodine quantitation by means of XRF, particular attention being paid to the sources of error affecting the precision and accuracy of the measurement.

## 2. MEASURING PROCEDURE

Intrathyroidal iodine quantitation is based on the assumption, well verified in practical conditions, that the quantity of iodine (mg) present in the irradiated volume of the neck is proportional to the intensity of the iodine $K\alpha$ photopeak, i.e., to the net counting rate in the $K\alpha$ discrimination window (Fig. 1).

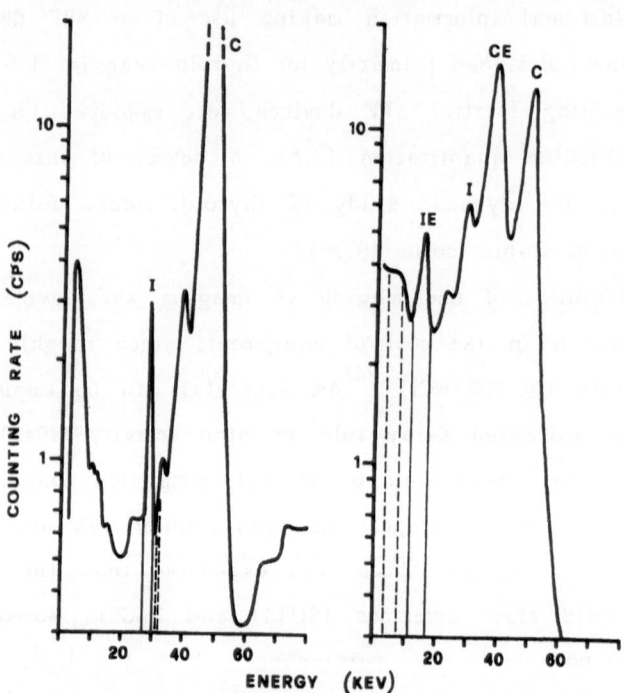

FIGURE 1. Energy spectra collected by means of a HpGe detector (left; adapted from ref. (11)) and a Kr-gas counter (right; adapted from ref. (10)) on neck-thyroid phantoms at iodine concentrations comparable with that in normal thyroid. C = Compton scatter peak; I = iodine $K\alpha$ peak; CE = Compton "escape" peak (Compton energy minus Kr-$K\alpha$ fluorescence energy); IE = iodine "escape" peak (iodine $K\alpha$ minus Kr-$K\alpha$). Possible choices of the $K\alpha$ window (continuous vertical lines) and the background window (dashed lines) are indicated.

Background due to source radiation scattered by the neck tissues is usually determined by selecting a window outside the photopeak (Fig. 1). The ratio (r) between the counting rate ($R_{bw}$) in the background window and the background counting rate ($R_b$) in the Kα window is determined on a tissue equivalent phantom of the neck in which no iodine is present:

$$r = R_b/R_{bw} \qquad \text{(neck phantom without iodine)} \qquad (1)$$

Provided the background window is chosen in the low energy part of the spectrum, as indicated in Figure 1, the ratio r is only very slightly affected by variations in the shape and internal geometry of the neck.

The net counting rate ($R_I$) is determined from $R_{bw}$ and the total counting rate (R) in the iodine Kα window:

$$R_I = R - r R_{bw} \qquad (2)$$

The iodine quantity (I) is then given by

$$I = k R_I \qquad (3)$$

where k is a constant to be evaluated by calibration of the measuring system, i.e., by determining $R_I$ in at least one condition in which the iodine quantity I is known. However, due to the low energy of the fluorescence X-rays from iodine (28.5 KeV, half thickness in soft tissue ≃ 20 mm), k can be considered constant only if the measuring geometry is strictly invariable, i.e., fixed external shape of the neck, fixed dimensions and location of the trachea, and fixed distribution of thyroidal iodine. Thus a value of k would have to be determined for each subject since the above-mentioned geometric parameters vary considerably from one subject to another. However, since this is not practical, gross approximations are usually made in the calibration procedure. k is estimated with reference to an "average" geometric configuration of the neck and thyroid, making use of tissue equivalent phantoms.

A slight modification to this procedure, proposed by Palmer et al. (2), consists in a double calibration on phantoms representing two classes of subjects, lean and obese. However, classification of subjects, e.g., based upon palpation of the neck, is subjective and thus not reliable.

## 3. MEASURING PRECISION AND ACCURACY

### 3.1. Precision

Random errors due to the statistical fluctuations of the counts will determine the precision of the measurement which is inversely related to the standard deviation ($\sigma_I$) of the estimated iodine quantity.

It is easy to demonstrate from the above equations that the relative precision increases, i.e., the ratio $\sigma_I/I$ decreases, as the background ratio (r) decreases. Thus, from eq. (1), $R_{bw}$ should be as wide as possible. However, in practice, the value of r is not usually less than about 1, due to limitations in the choice of the background window.

In order to evaluate the influence of other parameters on the measuring precision, an expression of the relative standard deviation was derived from eqs. (2) and (3). If we assume r = 1 and infinite measuring accuracy, i.e., no errors affecting the estimate of k, we have

$$\frac{\sigma_I}{I} = \frac{\sigma_{R_I}}{R_I} = \frac{1}{R_I} \left( \frac{R_I + 2 R_{bw}}{T} \right)^{\frac{1}{2}} \tag{4}$$

where T is the counting time.

The net counting rate can be approximately expressed in terms of the main measuring parameters as

$$R_I = \alpha \, \varepsilon_i \, \varepsilon_g \, \phi \tag{5}$$

where $\alpha$ is a proportionality constant which includes the tissue absorption effect, $\varepsilon_i$ and $\varepsilon_g$ are the intrinsic and geometric detection efficiencies, respectively, and Ø is the source photon flux. Thus, eq. (4) can be rewritten as

$$\frac{\tilde{\sigma}_I}{I} = \left( \frac{1 + \frac{2}{SNR}}{\alpha \, \varepsilon_i \, \varepsilon_g \, \emptyset \, T} \right)^{\frac{1}{2}} \tag{6}$$

where SNR (= $R_I/R_{bw}$) is the signal to noise ratio which depends on the energy resolution of the detector.

Equation (6) indicates that the precision increases with the integrated flux (ØT), i.e., with the absorbed dose. A four-fold increase in the integrated flux leads to a two-fold increase in precision. Moreover, since the counting time T should be as short as possible, a relatively high photon flux is needed, the limitations being the dead-time and pile-up effects. Optimization of the electronics, e.g., decrease in the shaping time, enables a higher photon flux to be used without impairing the detector performances.

The characteristics of the detector are described in eq. (6) by the parameters $\varepsilon_i$, $\varepsilon_g$ and SNR. Typical values of the intrinsic efficiency ($\varepsilon_i$) at the energy of 28.5 KeV are 100%, 70% and 30% for the HpGe, Si(Li) and Kr-gas detectors, respectively. The geometric efficiency ($\varepsilon_g$), at constant iodine distribution, is proportional to the area of the detector entrance window which should, therefore, be as wide as possible (eq. (6)), even if this generally implies a slight decrease in the energy resolution of the detector. 500 mm$^2$ is a typical value of the useful detection area for the above-mentioned detectors. However, it should be borne in mind that Kr-gas counters with an entrance window four-fold greater are available. Finally, in real measuring conditions on a normal subject the SNR has a value of about 2 for the HpGe and Si(Li) detectors, and about 0.2 for the Kr-gas counter, due to the different energy resolution (Fig. 1).

With these values for the main parameters, the precision (eq. (6)) is comparable for HpGe and Si(Li), while it is decreased about four-fold with the Kr-gas counter. Thus, a 4-5% precision for a Kr-gas counter, a value which has been obtained in practical conditions (10), corresponds to about 1% for a solid state detector, at the same photon flux and counting time.

## 3.2. Accuracy

As stated in Section 2, the value of k (eq. (3)) varies when the measuring geometry changes with respect to the calibration geometry. This leads to a systematic error (calibration error) in each subject, thus affecting the accuracy of the measurement.

If a series of subjects is considered, the calibration error varies, with a certain unknown distribution, depending on the deviation of the effective neck-thyroid geometry in each subject with respect to the calibration geometry.

"A priori" evaluation of the calibration errors is difficult since several geometric parameters, pertaining to both the neck and the thyroid, affect the result. However, some indications can be obtained if, as a first approximation, only the mean depth of the thyroid is considered variable, while the neck geometry and the size, shape and orientation of the gland are assumed to be invariable.

A decrease in the net counting rate $(R_I)$ at increasing mean depth $(D)$ of the thyroid may then be expected, due to the tissue absorption of both the excitation $\gamma$-rays and the fluorescence X-rays:

$$R_I(D) = R_{I0} \, e^{-(\mu_1 + \mu_2) \, D} \tag{7}$$

where $\mu_1 = 0.020 \text{ mm}^{-1}$ and $\mu_2 = 0.035 \text{ mm}^{-1}$ are the total linear absorption coefficients in soft tissue and the energies of 60 KeV and 28.5 KeV, respectively.

The theoretical pattern of eq. (7) is compared in Figure 2 with the experimental curve obtained on phantoms making use of a [241]Am source with a wide angle collimator. As can be seen, the experimental curve is still monoexponential but it is far steeper than

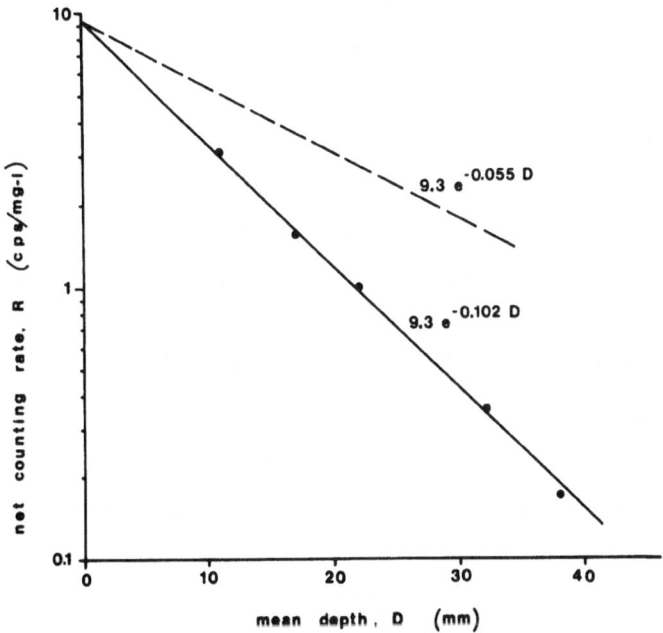

FIGURE 2. Theoretical (upper curve) and experimental (lower curve) variation of the net counting rate with mean depth of the thyroid. An Am-241 source with a wide angle collimator and a cylindrical lobe phantom (8 mm inner diameter) embebbed in a scatter medium were used in the experimental arrangement.

the theoretical curve. This is due to two geometric effects: i) the mean solid angle, useful for detecting the fluorescence X-rays, decreases at increasing depth of the thyroid; ii) the primary photon flux which irradiates the thyroid decreases at increasing depth since the $\gamma$-beam is divergent. This last effect is minimized if a straight bore collimator is employed, as is usual in fluorescent scanners equipped with an X-ray tube. An exponential coefficient equal to 0.087 mm$^{-1}$ was obtained in the same experimental conditions as those in Figure 2 but making use of a straight bore collimator 1 cm in length.

Furthermore, another effect should be mentioned, i.e., the enhancement of the fluorescence due to radiation scattered towards the thyroid by the surrounding tissues. This effect was investigated by comparing the counts obtained on small thyroid phantoms, placed at varying distances from the detector, with and without a scatter medium around them. Results show that, unless the diffusion effect contributes markedly to the excitation of the iodine fluorescence (20-30%), its dependence on the depth of the thyroid is very slight both with the wide angle and the straight bore collimators.

In summary, the net counting rate decreases with the mean depth of the thyroid according to a monoexponential function the coefficient of which is greater than $0.055$ $mm^{-1}$ and can rise to about $0.1$ $mm^{-1}$ at increasing divergence of the primary photon beam. Thus, from eq. (7), the variation in the net counting rate, per millimeter change in mean depth of the thyroid, falls within the limits:

$$5.5 \ \%/mm < \frac{1}{R_{10}} \ \frac{dR_I}{dD} \ \stackrel{\sim}{<} \ 10 \ \%/mm$$

Since the mean depth of the gland may vary from one subject to another by as much as several millimeters, the consequent error is very high and far greater than that due to random errors (Section 3.1.). It may therefore be concluded that the main problem in XRF quantitation of intrathyroidal iodine is accuracy rather than precision. Thus the development of an adequate calibration procedure is more important than the use of sophisticated and expensive instrumentation with high quality performances.

## 4. DEPTH SCANNING: A POSSIBLE TOOL TO IMPROVE ACCURACY

### 4.1. Calibration method and measuring procedure

In order to improve the accuracy in XRF intrathyroidal iodine quantitation, the distribution in depth of the iodine should be taken into account either by "a posteriori" correction or by an adequate "a priori" calibration of the measuring system. Our latest investigations have focused on this second alternative.

As far as the calibration model is concerned, each lobe of the thyroid is considered as 5 slices, as shown in Figure 3, and the un-

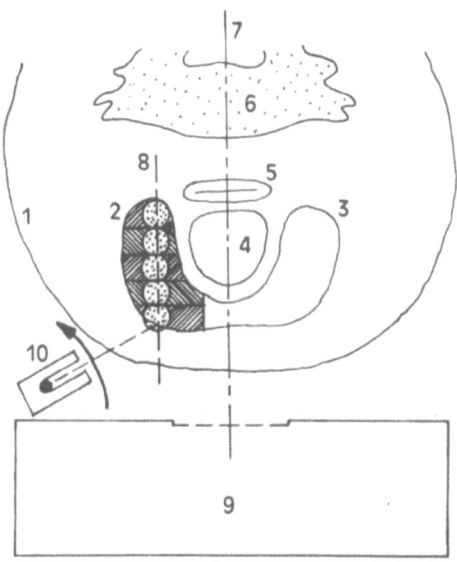

FIGURE 3. Schematic drawing of the neck section and calibration model for a single lobe. 1, neck surface; 2 and 3, right and left thyroid lobe, respectively; 4, trachea; 5, esophagus; 6, cervical vertebra; 7, neck axis; 8, calibration axis; 9, Kr-gas proportional counter; 10, rotating Am-241 sources (4x15 mCi) and collimator assembly. The dashed areas represent an ideal division of the lobe into slices. The round dotted areas are the corresponding "lobe pixels" of fixed height in which, for calibration purposes, the iodine content of each slice is considered concentrated.

known iodine content of each slice is regarded as concentrated in one cylindrical "lobe pixel", 8 mm inner diameter and 35 mm in length.

The source-collimator assembly rotates around a vertical axis parallel to the neck surface (Fig. 3), thus permitting "depth scanning" of the neck. The other side of the neck is scanned in a similar way making use of a second identical source-collimator assembly (not shown in Figure 3). The net counting rate is recorded at each angular step of about 3° and then plotted against the distance (d) between the intercept of the beam axis with the calibration axis and the neck surface ("depth scanning profile").

Calibration is performed on phantoms (Fig. 4) by recording the depth scanning profiles on a standard lobe pixel placed at 5 contiguous distances (D) from the neck surface. Each profile (Fig. 5) is then fitted with the gaussian function:

$$R_{I,i}(d) = R_{I,i}^* \; exp \left\{ - \frac{4 \; ln2 \left[d - (D_i + \Delta D_i)\right]^2}{W_i^2} \right\} \qquad (i = 1,\ldots,5) \quad (8)$$

where $R_{I,i}^*$ is the maximum counting rate, $\Delta D_i$ is the shift of the position of the maximum with respect to the center of the lobe pixel and $W_i$ is the width at half maximum of the gaussian curve. The maximum counting rate for each position of the lobe pixel is proportional to the iodine content of the pixel, i.e.,

$$R_{I,i}^* = k_i \; I_i \qquad\qquad\qquad (9)$$

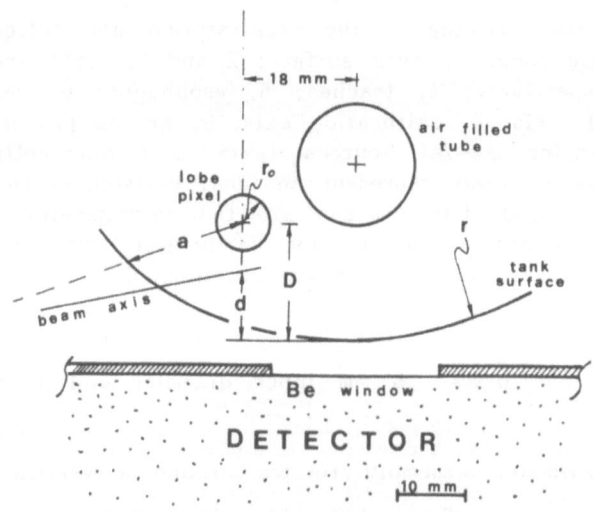

FIGURE 4. Schematic drawing of the calibration phantom. Distance (d) of the beam axis intercept from the neck surface and mean depth (D) of the lobe pixel are variable. The neck phantom is a cylindrical tank of plexiglass filled with water. The lobe pixel is a cylindrical tube of plexiglass ($r_o$ = 4 mm; height 35 mm) filled with an iodine water solution (5000 ppm; iodine content 8.8 mg). Supports and screws (not shown) are in nylon.

where the $k_i$ (i= 1,..,5) are calibration constants the values of which are given by the experimental curve in Figure 2.

The depth scanning profile on the entire thyroid lobe is given approximately by the sum of the contributions from the 5 lobe pixels. Thus, from eqs. (8) and (9), we have

$$R_I(d) = \sum_{i=1}^{5} R_{I,i} = \sum_{i=1}^{5} \left\{ k_i \exp\left[ - \frac{4 \ln2 \ (d-D_i - \Delta D_i)^2}{W_i^2} \right] \right\} I_i$$

In this equation, the values of $k_i$, $\Delta D_i$ and $W_i$ are derived from the above-described calibration. Thus, the iodine content $(I_i)$ of each lobe pixel, at distance $D_i$ from the neck surface, can be calculated with a best-fit procedure on the basis of the measured values of $R_I$. The unweighted least squares method was used.

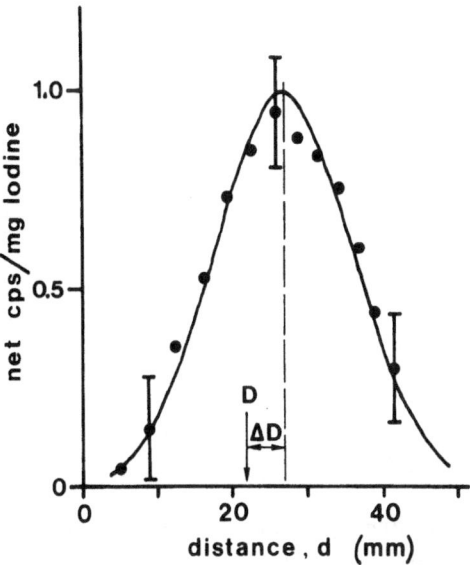

FIGURE 5. Typical depth scanning profile determined on a lobe pixel. For key to symbols see Figure 4. Continuous line is the best-fit gaussian function.

78

## 4.2. Validation tests

In order to assess the validity of this method, several tests were performed on phantoms of a single thyroid lobe in various geometrical arrangements. A typical example is given in Figure 6 which shows the analysis of measurements performed on the same lobe phantom at three different inclinations with respect to the neck surface.

Results of the tests showed good agreement between the effective iodine content, kept constant at 10.2 mg, and the calculated values

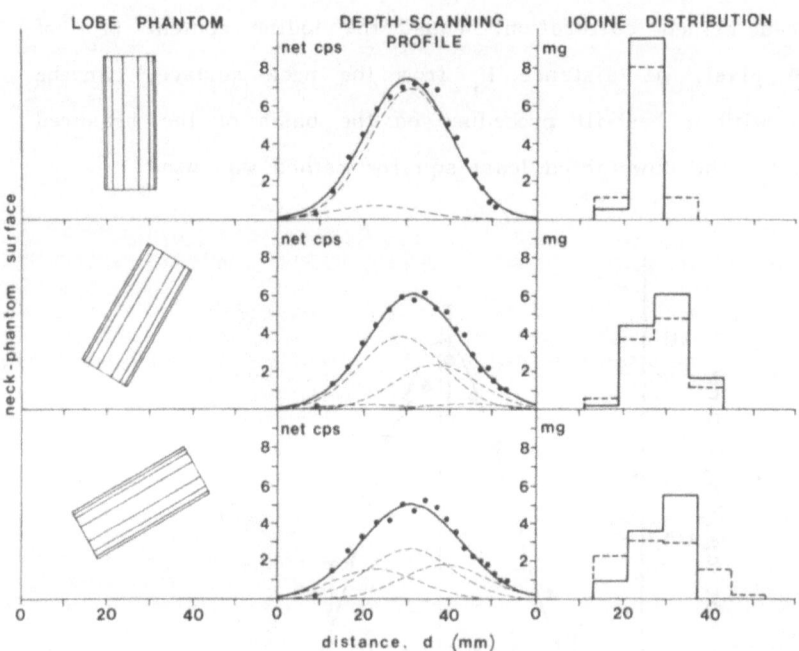

FIGURE 6. Left: different arrangements of the same lobe phantom (inner diameter 12 mm; iodine content 10.2 mg) within the neck phantom. Center: corresponding depth scanning profiles obtained by rotation of the source–collimator assembly (see text); continuous lines are the best-fit curves; dashed lines represent the components due to each lobe pixel. Right: effective and calculated depth distributions of iodine (dashed and continuous lines, respectively).

Table 1. Phantom tests (10.2 mg of iodine in a cylindrical phantom of one thyroid lobe)

| Geometrical arrangement | | | Maximum net counting rate (cps) | Calculated iodine content (mg) |
|---|---|---|---|---|
| Mean depth (mm) | Inclination (0°=vertical) | Diameter (mm) | | |
| 26 | 0° | 12 | 7.2 | 9.9 |
| 28 | 30° | 12 | 6.1 | 12.0 |
| 28 | 60° | 12 | 5.2 | 10.2 |
| 24 | 0° | 12 | 9.4 | 10.5 |
| 30 | 0° | 12 | 6.0 | 9.9 |
| 36 | 0° | 12 | 3.6 | 10.7 |
| 24 | 0° | 8 | 5.3 | 7.2 |
| 24 | 0° | 12 | 7.1 | 9.9 |
| 24 | 0° | 20 | 6.4 | 11.6 |
| mean $\pm$ 1 SD | | | 6.3 $\pm$ 1.6 | 10.2 $\pm$ 1.4 |
| 100 SD/mean | | | 26% | 13% |

(Table 1). It is worthwhile pointing out that the standard deviation of the calculated iodine content was much lower than that of the maximum counting rate (13% vs 26%), thus suggesting that with the proposed method a marked improvement in accuracy could be obtained with respect to methods based on calibration with phantoms of a "normal thyroid" in a fixed geometrical arrangement.

A preliminary study performed on one normal volunteer (Fig. 7) demonstrated the applicability of the proposed method "in vivo". However, in practice this scanning procedure and data elaboration would need to be completely automatic and in this respect micro-computerization of the system is at present under study in our laboratory.

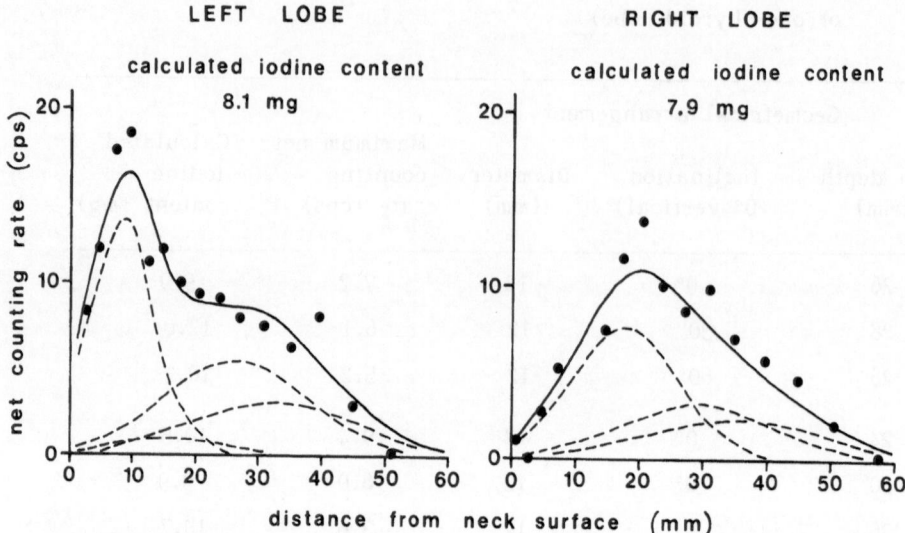

FIGURE 7. Example of depth scanning on each thyroid lobe of a normal volunteer. The best-fit curves and the components are represented with continuous and dashed lines, respectively. Counting time was 100 s for each point; the estimated dose absorbed by the thyroid was about 15 mrem.

## 5. CONCLUSIONS

The main problem in XRF iodine quantitation "in vivo" is the calibration of the measuring system, due to wide variations in the measuring geometry from one subject to another. The performances of the spectrometer used, particularly of the detector, are of minor importance unless an adequate calibration method is developed.

These considerations do not, however, apply to the determination of the iodine distribution (fluorescent image) since this is a relative measurement not requiring calibration.

From a practical point of view, the use of a Kr-gas counter and low activity [241]Am sources in a non-imaging system would cut equipment costs to an acceptable level ( < US$ 10,000). Moreover, unlike the XRF devices designed for thyroid imaging, a non-imaging device can be specifically optimized for intrathyroidal iodine quantitation. The depth scanning procedure described here is one possible approach in this direction.

ACKNOWLEDGEMENTS

The authors are grateful to Miss Adriana Shields for helpful advice in the preparation of the manuscript. This work is partly supported by Grant no. D.D.15.12.79/Cap.1572/Es.79, Ministero della Sanità.

REFERENCES

1. Patton JA, Hollifield JW, Brill AB, Lee GS, and Patton DD. 1976. Differentiation between malignant and benign solitary thyroid nodules by fluorescent scanning. J Nucl Med 17:17.
2. Palmer DW, Deconinck F, Swann SJ, Okerlund M, Kaufman L, Hoffer PB. 1976. Low cost intrathyroidal iodine quantitation with a fluorescent scanner. Radiology 119:733.
3. Thrall JH, Burman KD, Gillin MT, Corcoran RJ, Johnson MC, and Wartofsky L. 1977. Solitary autonomous thyroid nodules: comparison of fluorescent and pertechnetate imaging. J Nucl Med 18:1064.
4. Aubert B, Fragu P, Di Paola M, Rougier P, and Tubiana M. 1981. Application of X-ray fluorescence to the study of iodine distribution and content in the thyroid. Eur J Nucl Med 6:407.
5. Rougier P, Fragu P, Aubert B, Parmentier C, and Tubiana M. 1981. Mesure du contenu en iode intrathyroidien par fluorescence X: interet et applications. Path Biol 23:31.
6. Palmer DW, Kaufman L, and Deconinck F. 1979. Current developments in instrumentation for fluorescent scanning of the thyroid. In: Medical Applications of Fluorescent Excitation Analysis, Kaufman L & Price DC Eds, CRC Press, Boca Raton, Florida, USA, p. 139.
7. Gollnick DA, and Greenfield MA. 1978. The in vivo measurement of the total iodine content of the thyroid gland by X-ray fluorescence. Radiology 126:197.
8. Imamura K, Sasaki Y, Sekita N, Someya K, and Fujii M. 1979. Quantitative in vivo measurement of thyroidal iodine content by static X-ray fluorescence technique: some preliminary clinical observations. Invest Radiol 14:316.
9. Pavoni P, Frazzoli FV, and Magrini A. 1976. Radioisotope X-ray fluorescence technique in the dynamic study of thyroid behaviour under iodine load. Eur J Nucl Med 1:117.
10. Magrini A, Di Luzio S, Izzo G, and Raganella L. 1982. Intra-thyroidal iodine determination by X-ray fluorescence. In: X-Ray Fluorescence (XRF & PIXE) in Medicine, Cesareo R Ed, Field Educational Italia, Acta Medica, Rome, Italy, p. 87.
11. Patton JA, and Brill AB. 1978. Simultaneous emission and fluorescent scanning of the thyroid. J Nucl Med 19:464.

VI  QUALITY-CONTROL PROCEDURES AND EVALUATION OF A FLUORESCENT
THYROID SCANNER

H.W. WAHNER, M.D.


1.  INTRODUCTION

A few years ago we had the opportunity of evaluating a
commercial fluorescent scanning instrument and of using it for
thyroid imaging and quantitation.  With this instrument, we
were able to obtain clinically satisfactory and state-of-the-
art iodine quantitation in the thyroid gland and iodine distribution images.  To learn more about the method, we evaluated the
effect of various factors that could conceivably influence the
measurements.  These observations and the clinical results have
been published (1-3).  The objective of this review is to summa-
rize these observations and attempt to define various quality-
control experiments that could be performed with each system
before appropriate interpretation of results is made.  All
observations made here are valid only for a system that is of a
design similar to the one used in this study, and a different
approach may be necessary when different designs are utilized.

Critical factors that should be considered in the evaluation of a fluorescence thyroid scanner and that are important
for an understanding of the function are (1) the selection of
an appropriate background region within the energy spectrum,
(2) the mode of background subtraction, and (3) an assessment
of the limitations for imaging and quantitation due to a given
detector-source geometry.  These factors will be treated in
the following presentation, along with pitfalls one may encounter in interpreting clinically useful thyroid images.

2.  METHODS AND PROCEDURES

2.1.  Description of the instrument

The system used in this study was a Kevex Scan II thyroid
fluorescent scanner adapted to a Picker Magna-Scanner II.  In
this instrument the excitation beam is produced by a collimated
10-Ci $^{241}$Am source (59.7 keV).  The collimator is a double-
focused multihole collimator providing an intrinsic resolution
of 7 mm.  The detector is not collimated and is in a satellite
position at a 30-degree angle.  The physical appearance of the
instrument and the source-detector design are illustrated in
Figures 1 and 2, respectively.  The detector system in the
instrument was a high-resolution, silicon-lithium drifted
semiconductor with an active area of 500 mm$^2$.  The electronic
components are schematically presented in Figure 3.

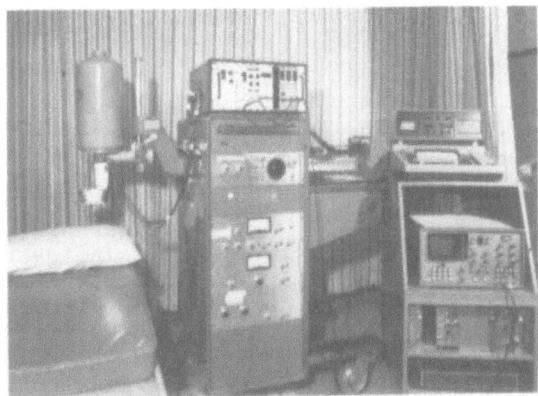

FIGURE 1.  Kevex thyroid fluorescence instrument attached
to a Picker Magna-Scanner with multichannel analyzer.
Patient's bed is to the left.  (From ref. 2 by permission.)

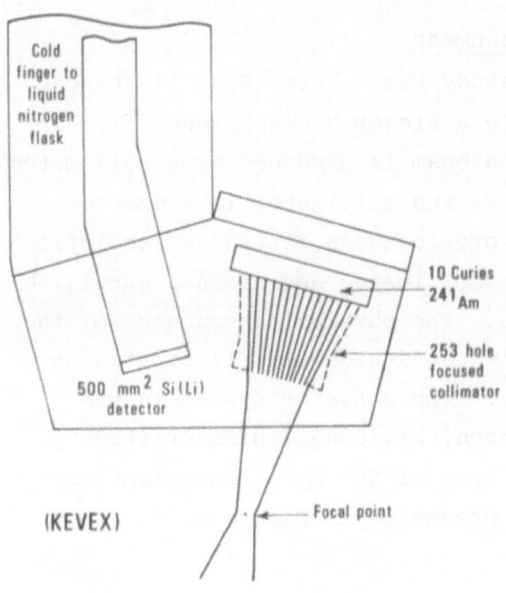

FIGURE 2. Source detector design of thyroid fluorescence scanner. Si(Li) = silicon-lithium. (From ref. 2 by permission.)

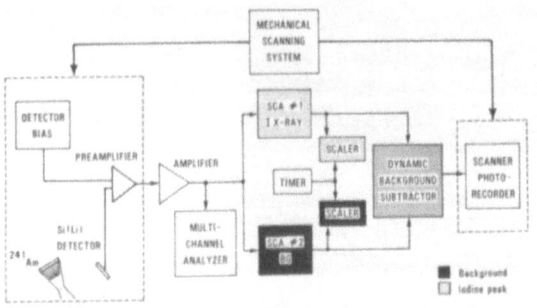

FIGURE 3. Schematic presentation of the electronic components of a thyroid fluorescence scanning system. SCA = single-channel analyzer; Si(Li) = silicon-lithium; BG = background; I = iodine. (From ref. 2 by permission.)

Components of such a system are an amplifier, a multi-channel analyzer, two single-channel analyzers, two scalers, timers, and the dynamic background subtraction module (Kevex model 4840). The dynamic subtraction module produces a signal equivalent to the difference of the count rates from two single-channel analyzers, set to represent an energy window over the $K_\alpha$ iodine x-ray peak and the background region.  The output from this system was put into a multichannel analyzer. An energy spectrum obtained with the fluorescence scanner (59.7-keV $^{241}$Am excitation source) from the thyroid gland of a normal subject is shown in Figure 4.

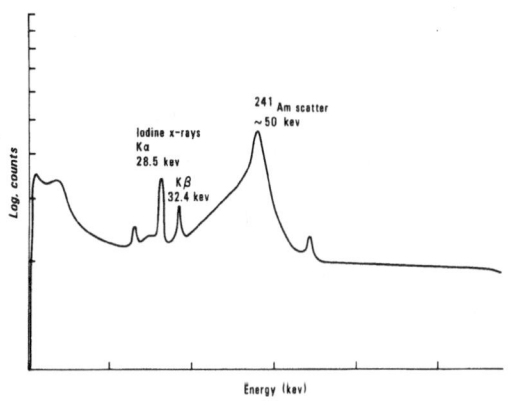

FIGURE 4.  Energy spectrum.  The spectrum shows the characteristic x-rays of iodine--$K_\alpha$ at 28.5 keV, $K_\beta$ at 32.4 keV--in close proximity to the very prominent scatter peak from the americium source. The $K_\beta$ peak of the characteristic iodine x-ray is in immediate proximity to the americium scatter peak and is altered by it.  Another scatter peak, somewhat lower than the $K_\beta$ peak, can also be noted. (From ref. 2 by permission.)

The angular relationship of the excitation beam and the detector affects the energy of the Compton scatter peak, which is the major peak in the fluorescence energy spectrum.  As the angle reaches a maximum of 180 degrees, the Compton scatter peak has a minimum energy value and the iodine peak and scatter peak are closest together.  A minimum intensity (or height) of the scatter peak is found at a source-detector angle of 90 degrees.  The energy resolution that can be obtained with modern solid-state detectors, however, is such that these considerations are not limiting factors in actual instrument design.  Of importance, however, is that a focusing effect is created.  For this, the 90-degree angle would be unsuitable. A compromise used in one commercial instrument employed here is a detector-source angle of 30 degrees, resulting in an effective scatter angle of 150 degrees.

Window settings with this instrument included a window
around the 28.5 $K_\alpha$ x-ray. The $K_\beta$ x-ray at 32.4 keV was re-
jected for counting because of the predominance of scatter
events and the degree of slope in this region. For background
subtraction (ideally counts equivalent to the count rate in
the $K_\alpha$ window when no iodine is present), an energy window
between 19.3 and 22.2 keV was selected. This region in the
spectrum was selected on the basis of the absence of slope and
the equivalence to the count rate in the iodine window under
varying experimental scatter conditions (details follow).

Measurements were made at constant distances of 2.5 cm
between probe and skin surface. Scan speed of 25 cm/min and
line spacing of 0.3 cm were used, which allowed the thyroid
gland to be scanned within 20 minutes. The events selected
to be recorded on film and used for iodine quantitation were
the net events occurring in the $K_\alpha$ x-ray window.

## 2.2. Subjects and tissue-equivalent phantoms

Thyroid glands of normal subjects were scanned, and iodine
quantitation was performed. Studies were also performed with
a standard Picker thyroid phantom containing hot and cold
areas (varying concentrations of potassium iodide) and different activities in the two lobes. A special phantom was made
by pouring hot gelatin made up with different concentrations
of potassium iodide into plastic Petri dishes. Nodules were
represented by plastic cylinders inserted into the gelatin
and filled with water and having different concentrations of
potassium iodide. Care was taken to avoid leakage into the
gelatin (Fig. 5).

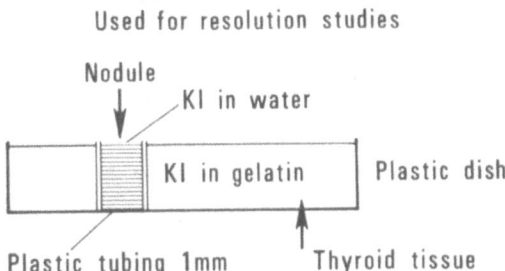

THYROID PHANTOM
Used for resolution studies

FIGURE 5. Schematic representation of a phantom to study performance characteristics of thyroid fluorescence system, particularly resolution studies.

## 3. RESULTS

### 3.1. Evaluation of proper background selection

The proper background has to be found empirically by study of the spectrum under varying conditions. This was performed in a series of three experiments. First, two athyroid patients were scanned over the neck region. The count rates obtained from the iodine $K_\alpha$ peak window and the background window differed by +4.5 and -1.5%. Significantly greater differences were found when other regions of the spectrum were selected as background. Second, energy spectra were obtained from a normal control subject at three locations in the anterior neck region. The results are illustrated in Figure 6.

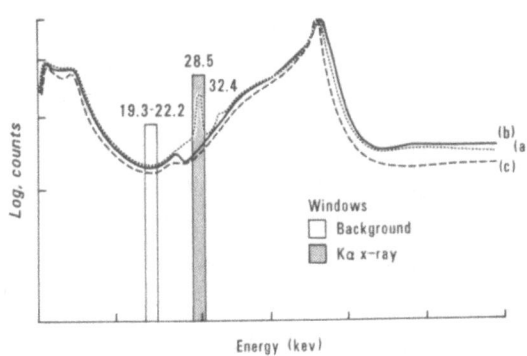

FIGURE 6. Energy spectra obtained from normal control subject. Curve a was obtained over thyroid gland, curve b over trachea above thyroid gland, and curve c over lateral region of neck outside thyroid region. Energy windows selected for $K_\alpha$ iodine x-ray and representative background are shown. (From ref. 2 by permission.)

Curve a was obtained over the thyroid gland, curve b over the trachea above the thyroid gland, and curve c over the lateral region of the neck outside the thyroid region. The energy windows selected for the $K_\alpha$ iodine x-ray and for background are shown. Differences noted in these spectra are due to the presence or absence of iodine (see peak in curve a only over the thyroid gland), the amount of scattering material within the beam path, and the beam-detector response to source distance (curvature of thyroid). The spectrum obtained over the thyroid gland demonstrates the peak corresponding to the $K_\alpha$ (28.5 keV) and $K_\beta$ (32.4 keV) iodine x-rays. Again, the most prominent peak, however, is the Compton scatter peak of the 59.7-keV americium gamma radiation. During a thyroid fluorescent scan, far less than 1% of the total counts are registered in the iodine region; with a technetium scan this figure is 20 to 30%, and it is even higher with an $^{131}$I scan. The spectra obtained outside the thyroid gland show the absence of iodine but a slightly different scatter pattern. The energy window set at 19.3 to 22.2 keV is placed at a valley of the spectrum and at a site where the three spectra do not differ significantly. Close inspection of the three spectra inside the background window shows that the background is not constant as the scanning beam traverses the thyroid gland from curve c (lateral neck) to curve a (thyroid) to curve b (midline, trachea) and then to a and back to c. This suggests that a constant background as used in some equipment should not be used and that the dynamic background subtraction method is superior. Third, the effect of an increased stable iodine background was demonstrated on images only. Quantitative determination of iodine was not possible with reliable accuracy under these circumstances (Fig. 7). In this case a patient had a standard technetium scan (a) for a large, palpable, firm nodule in the right lobe. An excretory urogram was performed 1 day later. The fluorescent scan (b) was performed about 30 minutes after completion of the urogram. The spectrum showed a small iodine $K_\alpha$ peak in the neck background. The image shows the high background in the tissue. However, the thyroid gland could be imaged with the essential information still visible. This information would not have been possible with $^{99m}$Tc or $^{131}$I scintigrams.

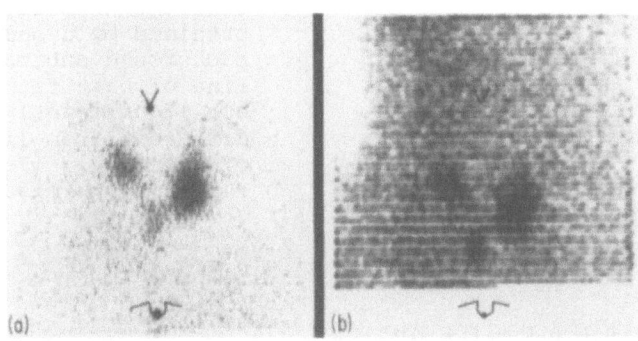

FIGURE 7. $^{99m}$TcO$_4$ scan (a) before an excretory urogram. The fluorescent scan (b) was performed about 30 minutes after the urogram. (From ref. 1 by permission.)

## 3.2. Selection of proper background subtraction mode

After selection empirically of the energy window for the background, a constant or dynamic background subtraction mode should be considered next. In the case of a constant background subtraction, a point outside the thyroid gland is chosen as background and then subtracted from each count from the specific iodine window. The dynamic background subtraction technique continuously monitors the count rate from the iodine minus the background window. For both modes, the background region has to be found empirically. Arguments in favor of the dynamic background subtraction mode have already been presented in the preceding paragraph. As a test of the effectiveness of the dynamic background subtraction module, the net count sum obtained by separate scalers was compared with the counts obtained by the dynamic subtraction module. Results are shown in Figure 8.

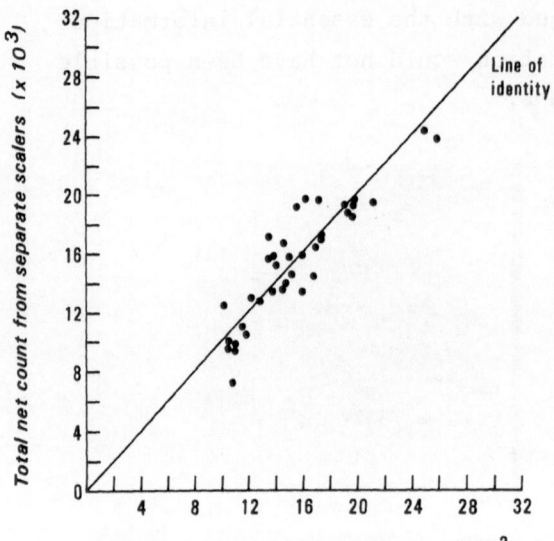

FIGURE 8. Plot of data comparing total count result obtained by separately scaling background and iodine counts with total count obtained by dynamic background subtraction. Line of best fit was not significantly different from line of identity. (From ref. 2 by permission.)

The line of best fit calculated by least-squares regression was not significantly different from the line of identity. This attests to the proper function of the dynamic background module. An excess in background subtraction would have resulted in an intercept that was significantly below zero.

The effect of the dynamic background subtraction technique on the thyroid images was evaluated by assessing its effect on the average information density, scan contrast, and count variations. This was calculated for scans on patients with high, normal, and low content of thyroid iodine. The results are summarized in Table 1. The results show that when any of the two background subtraction modes was used, average information density decreased but scan contrast and count variation increased. On subjective review of the scans, thyroid scans of subjects with normal iodine content showed only marginal improvement when background subtraction was used. This improvement was, however, significant when thyroid glands with low iodine content were scanned.

Table 1. Comparison of calculated imaging characteristics by means of dynamic background subtraction (DBS) and iodine peak only (I).

| Thyroid iodine content | Total scan counts | | | Average information density* | | Scan contrast† | | Scan count variation, %‡ | |
|---|---|---|---|---|---|---|---|---|---|
| | I | Back-ground | DBS | I | DBS | I | DBS | I | DBS |
| High | 46,305 | 26,833 | 19,907 | 264 | 113 | 0.86 | 1.0 | 0.5 | 1.4 |
| Normal | 34,106 | 23,596 | 11,855 | 223 | 77 | 0.78 | 1.0 | 0.5 | 2.0 |
| Low | 26,109 | 23,863 | 2,947 | 169 | 19 | 0.31 | 1.0 | 0.6 | 7.6 |

*Average information density = $\dfrac{\text{counts for complete scan}}{\text{scan speed x line space x time}}$.

†Scan contrast = $\dfrac{\text{count rate maximum-count rate minimum}}{\text{count rate maximum}}$.

‡Count variation for iodine peak only = $I^{\frac{1}{2}}/I \times 100$ and count variation using dynamic background subtraction = $[(I + BKG)^{\frac{1}{2}}/(I-BKG)] \times 100$.

From McCormick MV, Wahner HW. 1978. Effect of background radiation change on measurements of iodine by x-ray fluorescence technique. J Nucl Med Technol 6:30-33. By permission of Society of Nuclear Medicine.

## 3.3. Alterations in background by contamination with other frequently used radioisotopes

Since fluorescent thyroid scans are often performed to evaluate further the findings initially obtained from a [99m]Tc-pertechnetate or sodium iodide scan, the effect of these radioisotopes on quantitation and imaging of iodine distribution was evaluated by x-ray fluorescence. Figure 9 shows the [99m]Tc spectrum with the source shutter of the instrument closed.

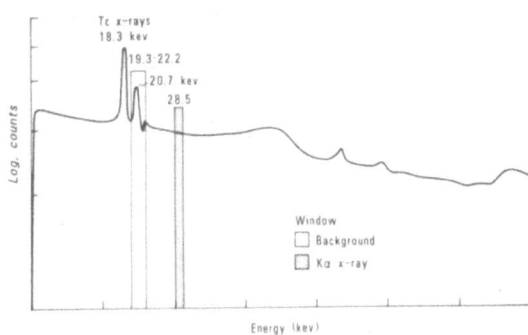

FIGURE 9. Energy spectrum of [99m]Tc obtained with fluorescence scanner with the excitation beam shutter closed. Characteristic x-rays of technetium are shown. (From ref. 2 by permission.)

The characteristic x-rays at 20.7 and 18.3 keV are seen. As can be noted, the 20.7-keV peak falls within the preselected background window, and the result is a high background signal.

Contamination of the thyroid or background resulted in falsely low imaging information and measurements of iodine quantitation. $^{99m}$Tc-pertechnetate in the thyroid phantom containing 30 mg of potassium iodide reduced the iodine quantitation by 0.4 mg iodine per microcurie present. Ten microcuries of $^{99m}$TcO$_4$ led to a significant loss of resolution of the image, and with 22 µCi, the outline of parts of the thyroid phantom was no longer recognizable.

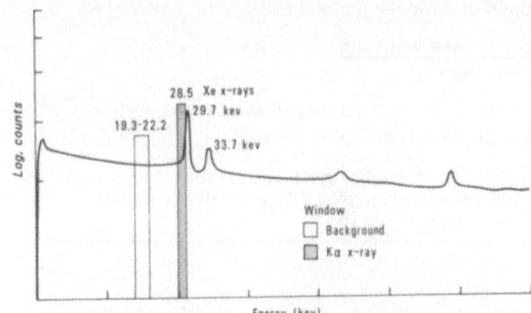

FIGURE 10. Energy spectrum of $^{131}$I obtained with fluorescence scanner with excitation beam shutter closed. Characteristic x-rays of xenon are shown. (From ref. 2 by permission.)

With sodium iodide ($^{131}$I) and the source shutter closed, the spectrum shows the characteristic xenon x-rays at 29.7 and 33.7 keV (Fig. 10). In this case the lower energy tail of the 29.7-keV peak falls within the $K_\alpha$ iodine x-ray window. This results in falsely high iodine quantitation and thyroid images. With the use of the same thyroid phantom as previously described, the addition of $^{131}$I falsely increased the quantitation by 0.3 mg of iodine per microcurie present. Images of the phantom showed poor resolution, particularly with respect to the recognition of the cold nodules.

In the case of gallium-67 backscatter from 93 keV, gamma emission falls into the background window to a greater proportion than into the $K_\alpha$ iodine window. This results in falsely low iodine quantitation. With 5 µCi of $^{67}$Ga added to the thyroid phantom, the original count rate was reduced by 50%, and with 13 µCi, only 1/10 of the counts was noted. The thyroid phantom image was significantly distorted with as little as 1.8 µCi of $^{67}$Ga added. With 20 µCi of $^{67}$Ga added, a scan suggesting the absence of iodine was obtained.

4.  LIMITATIONS DUE TO THE DETECTOR-SOURCE GEOMETRY

4.1.  Effect of overlying skin

The effect of overlying skin on the quantitation of iodine was evaluated by means of the Picker thyroid phantom filled with a potassium iodide solution.  Pig skin from a local butcher was packed on top of the phantom in layers from zero to 0.8 cm thickness.  Mean skin thickness of patients studied was 0.16 cm and ranged from 0.05 to 0.3 cm, as determined with skin calipers.

The results are illustrated in Figure 11.  Thickness of the skin is plotted against counts in milligrams of iodine in the tissue-equivalent phantom containing 5, 10, and 20 mg of iodine.  From a regression analysis $y = 992e^{-0.124x}$ and $r = -0.94$, where y is counts in milligrams of iodine and x is thickness of the overlying tissue in millimeters.  In practice, a factor for normal and for thick skin was used.

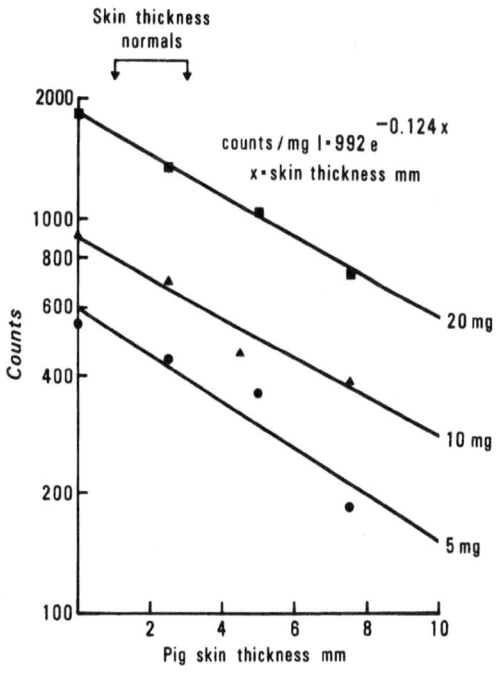

FIGURE 11.  Effect of skin thickness on iodine quantitation. (From ref. 1 by permission.)

## 4.2. Image distortion artifact

Because of the satellite position of the source relative to the detector and the curvature of the thyroid, an artifactual distortion of the image is introduced. This is illustrated in Figure 12. There is an asymmetry in the scan obtained from a circular phantom containing iodine on a curved surface. The image on the side of the excitation source appears more oval, smaller, and denser. The same artifact can be seen in a scan of a thyroid gland from a patient when the patient was scanned first in the usual position (Fig. 13a) and then rotated 180 degrees and re-scanned (Fig. 13b). The magnitude of this distortion varies with the design of the instrument. This effect should be considered when thyroid scans are interpreted for diagnostic purposes.

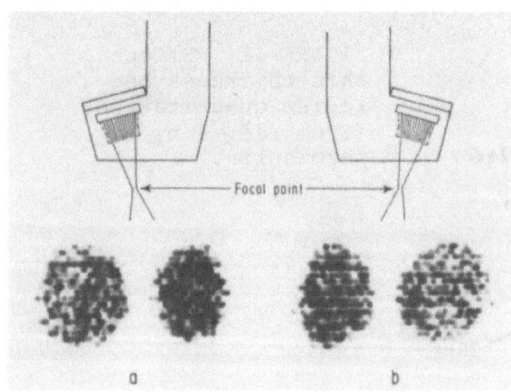

FIGURE 12. Example of image distortion artifact (see text).

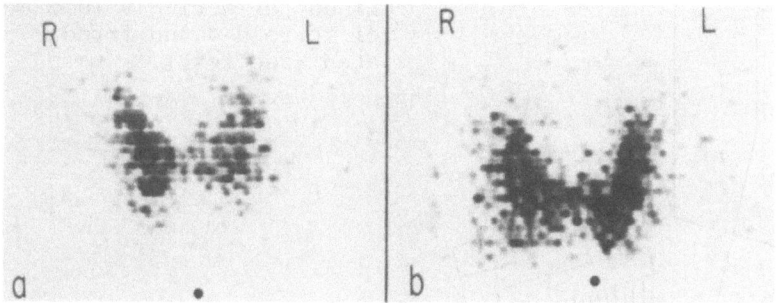

FIGURE 13.   Scan of thyroid gland in a patient (see text).

## 4.3.   Irradiated volume

The area in the target, here the thyroid gland, in which
fluorescence is generated depends on the geometric design of
the source and the detector.   In a single-source design with
source collimation, as used in our system, a sensitive volume
of the thyroid gland is irradiated at once.   Fluorescent
x-rays from this volume are seen by the detector.   The
efficiency of irradiation is, however, not the same in all
parts of the irradiated volume.   Isocount lines are shown in
Figure 14 for a region 2 to 4 cm away from the instrument
surface, the distance at which the thyroid gland is actually
scanned.   Given a thyroid gland of 1-cm thickness, measurements would be made within the 70% isocount range.   Changes
in thickness of the thyroid gland would affect the accuracy
of the measurement.   The volume of the target tissue
irradiated varies with the source-detector relationship.
With both source and detector collimation, the sensitive
volume could be reduced to be close to a point.   With this
design, a tomographic effect could be achieved.   However,
such a theoretic design has not found practical application.
When the volume was constant, such as in the gelatin phantom,
the count response to iodine concentration was linear over a
wide range (Fig. 15).   The lowest detectable iodine
concentration in water-filled phantoms was 0.1 mg/ml.

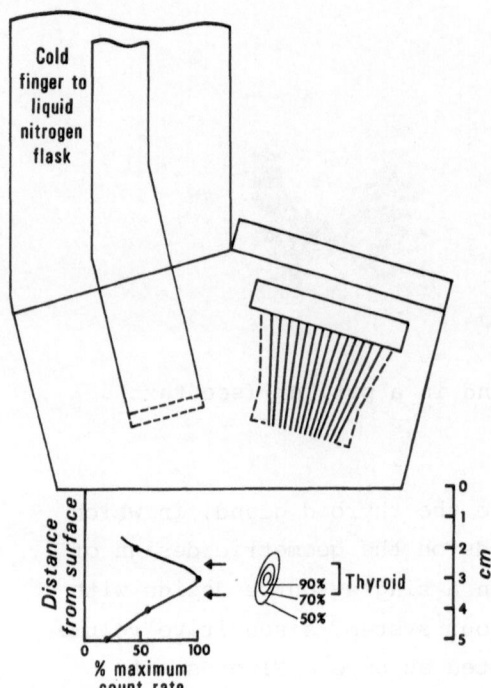

FIGURE 14. Isocount lines reflecting volume of thyroid gland irradiated (see text).

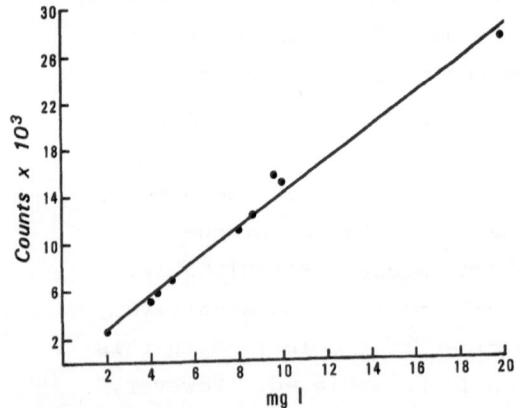

FIGURE 15. Iodine weight plotted against total count obtained by fluorescence scanning. Iodine as potassium iodide in solution was added to tissue-equivalent phantoms, and these were scanned by means of standard patient procedures. Measurements were performed in air. Distance from phantom to probe surface was 2.5 cm. From linear regression analysis: $y = 1,398x + 68$, $r = 0.99$, and $Sy \cdot x = \pm 913$, where y is total counts and x is amount of iodine (in milligrams) in phantom. (From ref. 1 by permission.)

## 4.4. Resolution

Perhaps the most important requirement of an instrument for thyroid scanning is its ability to detect small hypofunctioning (cold) nodules. This property depends not only on the actual site of the nodule but also on the ratio of activity within the hypofunctioning nodule and the surrounding tissue. This was tested with a phantom containing gelatin as tissue-equivalent material as previously described. The results are demonstrated in Table 2.

Table 2. Visualization of defects in gelatin phantoms.

| Concentration of iodide, mg/g gelatin | | Smallest defect, diameters (cm) |
|---|---|---|
| Matrix | 0.4 | |
| Defect | 0.0 | 0.7 |
| Matrix | 0.4 | |
| Defect | 0.2 | 1.5 |
| Matrix | 0.2 | |
| Defect | 0.0 | 2.1 |
| Matrix | 0.2 | |
| Defect | 0.1 | No visualization |

Under optimal conditions, a cold nodule of 0.7 cm could be detected in a thyroid gland that was normal with respect to iodine content. When compared with other imaging instruments at a similar level of nodule-to-background activity ($^{99m}$Tc), the gamma camera resolution (pin-hole collimator) was superior, but the resolution of the rectilinear scanner was about equal to that obtained with the thyroid fluorescence unit.

## 4.5. Reproducibility for long-range studies

For longitudinal studies in which changes over time are investigated, the instruments should have a good reproducibility. This factor was tested over a period of 4 months on a standard phantom containing 30 mg of iodide. With 72 measurements, the coefficient of variation (CV) was 8% of the mean. In three normal subjects scanned repeatedly

(10 to 24 times) the iodine content of the thyroid gland ranged between 15 and 25% (Table 3). In this experiment there was, however, no proof that the iodine content of the thyroid gland remained constant during this time.

Table 3. Reproducibility study.*

| Type of measurement | Subject | No. of times scanned | Total counts over thyroid | SD (counts) | CV (%) |
|---|---|---|---|---|---|
| Repeat measurement--same subject over 2 months | H | 9 | 10,306 | 977 | 9.48 |
| | A | 15 | 9,974 | 1,030 | 10.33 |
| Repeat measurement--same subject, same day | H | 4 | 10,750 | | 8.0 |
| | A | 4 | 9,525 | | 8.6 |

*Random counts without iodine source taken at multiple occasions showed a difference between counts in iodine and background channel of (±) 2.5%.

5. PITFALLS IN INTERPRETING THYROID FLUORESCENT IMAGES

Since the information obtained is derived from iodine regardless of its chemical properties, uptake in the neck is not necessarily associated with thyroid tissue. Positive scans suggesting ectopic thyroid tissue have been found in patients with contrast material from lymphangiography in lymph nodes in the neck (Fig. 16). This has been described in as brief a period as a few days (4) and as long as 2 years (3) after lymphangiography.

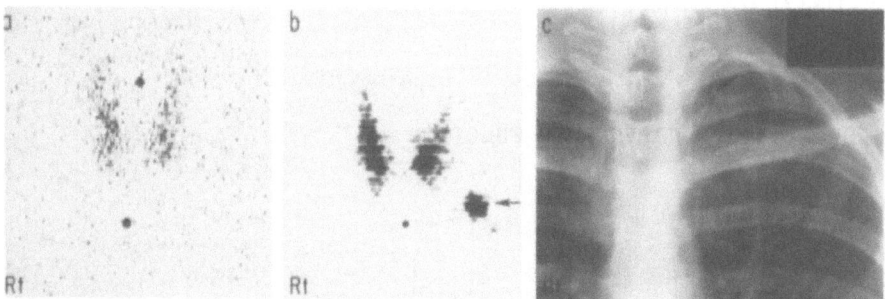

FIGURE 16. (a) Scintigram of thyroid gland made with $^{131}$I (NaI) with a 3-inch crystal, 19-hole collimator-detector. (b) Same thyroid scanned with the fluorescent scanner, show-ing ectopic thyroid tissue. (c) Radiography of anterior chest, showing subclavicular lymph node with contrast material (Lipiodol).

## ACKNOWLEDGMENT

The author wishes to acknowledge the help and technical expertise of Alan L. Orvis, Ph.D., Radiation Control Office at the Mayo Clinic, and Michael V. McCormick, B.S., technical associate at the time of the study. The help of the Kevex Corporation in providing the fluorescence system used in this investigation is appreciated. Part of this material was presented at the 24th Annual Meeting of the Society of Nuclear Medicine, Chicago, June 20-23, 1977.

## REFERENCES

1. Wahner HW, Sweet RA, McConahey WM, Duick DS. 1978. Fluorescent thyroid scanning: A method based on stable iodine measurements. Mayo Clin Proc 53:151-156.
2. McCormick MV, Wahner HW. 1978. Effect of background radiation change on measurements of iodine by x-ray fluorescence technique. J Nucl Med Technol 6:30-33.
3. Sweet RA, Wahner HW. 1977. False-positive fluorescence thyroid scan for ectopic thyroid tissue. J Nucl Med 18:1142-1143.
4. Nijensohn E, McCartney W, Hoffer PB. 1973. Identification of iodine in a supraclavicular lymph node following lymphography: A fluorescent scan artifact. J Nucl Med 14:179-180.

**PART II**: CLINICAL APPLICATIONS

VII STABLE IODINE AND THYROID FUNCTION

M.H. JONCKHEER

1. INTRODUCTION

The thyroid gland has a double specific role: iodine-dependent hormonogenesis and storage of iodine. The importance of the latter is reflected in the worldwide problem of endemic goiter due to inadequate iodine intake (01,02) and by the fact that iodine is present only in a few alimentary products and thus irregularly aivailable (03,04). Direct estimation of intrathyroidal iodine stores (ITI) in vivo in man was made possible by the introduction of the X-Ray-Fluorescence method (XRF) by Hoffer a few years ago (05); previously only indirect means were available, using radioactive iodine (06,07,08,09). It becomes thus possible to estimate in vivo in man the net effect of the storage function in an innocuous way allowing even repeated examinations with very acceptable radiation burdens. This technique can be used in routine clinical work as well as for more fundamental physiological studies (10). Three functional images of the thyroid can now be obtained in departments of nuclear medicine: one of iodine-trapping by means of radiopertechnetate, one of organification using radioiodine and one of iodine storage with XRF (11). The dissociation of these functions such as seen in goiter (12) can thus be demonstrated in these patients.

The total amount or the concentration of iodine (ITI conc) conditions overall thyroid function. This has repeatedly been shown directly in vivo in animal studies as well as in vitro, i.e. in cultured animal and human thyroid slices. Indirect evidence has been observed in vivo in man

(13). As quantifying ITI is possible with XRF, recent investigations with this technique allowed to demonstrate directly in man many facets of thyroid physiology, derived from animal studies and from indirect observations that were presumed to be related with the amount of stable iodine present in the human gland. It is the aim of the present review to recapitulate what is known about thyroid physiopathology, especially about stable iodine that is felt to be relevant to enlighten the results obtained in vivo in man by means of XRF.

## 2. NATURE OF INTRATHYROIDAL IODINE

Results obtained by means of XRF applied to the thyroid depend upon the stable iodine present and give information about its distribution and its amount. The technological problems involved that condition the reliability of these results are extensively discussed in Part I of this monograph and have been implicitly taken into account in what follows. It should be stressed however that no information at all can be gathered with this technique as to the nature of the iodine that one is measuring.

## 2. 1. Normal glands

In the normal human thyroid gland, the major form in which iodine is found consists of iodothyronines (triiodo-thyronine $T_3$, reverse triiodothyronine $rT_3$ and thyroxine $T_4$) and their precursors, the iodothyrosines (monoiodothyrosine MIT and diiodothyrosine DIT); about 20% is represented by other organic iodocompounds and inorganic iodine (14,03). The true proportion of each component is not exactly known because of the limitations of the analytical methods employed. Gross modifications of these proportions are well documented and the results of such investigations are relatively consistent.

Examples of normal values of total ITI (TITI) obtained by different methods in different parts of the world and at different periods, are represented in Tabel 1.

Table 1. Intrathyroidal iodine (ITI) in normal thyroid glands.

| REFERENCE | PLACE | | METHOD | T ITI mg | ITI conc. mg/gr |
|---|---|---|---|---|---|
| DeGroot et al. | U.S. | 1966 | RI | 11.2 | |
| Ermans et al. | Belgium | 1968 | NA | — | 0.62 ± 0.066 |
| Fisher et. al. | U.S. | 1969 | C | 15.0 | |
| Berson et al. | U.S. | 1969 | RI | 7.00 ± 10.0 | |
| Thilly et al. | Zaïre | 1973* | RI | 8.0 | |
| LeBlanc et al. | U.S. | 1973 | XRF** | — | 0.98 |
| Palmer et al. | U.S. | 1976 | XRF | 10.30 ± 2.2 | |
| | | | | 8.20 ± 2.5 | |
| Patton et al. | U.S. | 1976 | XRF | 10.70 ± 4.8 | |
| Thrall et al. | U.S. | 1978 | XRF | 10.50 ± 4.0 | |
| Hellstern et al. | Germany | 1978 | C | 17.13 ± 12.8 | 1.86 ± 10.50 |
| Nakashima et al. | Japan | 1978 | C | 7.70 ± 1.7 | |
| Wahner et al. | U.S. | 1978 | XRF | 15.50 ± 6.0 | |
| Okerlund et al. | U.S. | 1979 | XRF | 9.90 ± 6.0 | |
| Imamura et al. | Japan | 1979 | XRF | 10.60 ± 6.5 | |
| | | | | 17.60 ± 7.9 | |
| Leisner et al. | Germany | 1979 | XRF | — | 0.38 ± 0.070 |
| Rougier et al. | France | 1981 | XRF | 15.60 ± 4.8 | |
| Reinwein et al. | Germany | 1981 | C | 10.00 ± 2.3 | 0.325± 0.047 |
| Tadros et al. | G.B. | 1981 | XRF** | — | 1.03 ± 0.670 |
| Jonckheer et al. | Belgium | 1982 | XRF | 9.00 ± 3.7 | |

T ITI : total ITI
ITI conc. : ITI concentration
RI : indirect method using radioiodine
C : direct chemical method after exeresis
NA : neutron activation
XRF : X-Ray Fluorescence
* : one year after iodine supplementation
** : in vitro after exeresis

Other data concerning values in non-endemic and endemic goiter regions can be found in Delange and Ermans (02). The inspection of these data gives rise to some remarks relevant to the point in discussion. Some discordances are obvious, probably due to both methodological problems and the type of population investigated, but there is a certain agreement around 10-15 mg TITI in normal human subjects, as measured by kinetic analysis with radioiodine on the one hand and other methods on the other hand. As the first method measures total exchangeable iodine pool, it can be concluded that the XRF results reflect this pool. Ermans et al. (15) have shown that above a level of 0.250 mg I/gr thyroid tissue, there is no change in the relative proportion of iodocompounds in the thyroid and that there is a significant correlation between thyroglobulin iodination and iodine concentration in the gland. Furthermore, a correlation between the amount of thyroglobulin stored by each follicle and the degree of iodination of protein exists in normal glands (16). Thus in normal glands, the ITI represents an estimation of the amount of thyroid tissue present, sufficient to maintain euthyroidism.

A critical limit of TITI is therefore to be expected under which thyroid decompensation is met. This limit has not yet been defined for normal glands, but is had been suggested that it is situated around 2 to 3 mg in atrophic autoimmune thyroiditis (17,18). It is also apparent from published data (not shown in Table 1) that normal TITI values cover a wide range, the smallest range being reported in regions where iodine is supplemented in the diet. Although we have reported normal values to be 9 mg with a SD of 3.7 mg and considered TITI of 3 mg and 27 mg to be statistical outliers (10), we must admit that, as experience is accumulating, we encounter more patients with lower than normal TITI than the converse who do not present any other abnormality of their thyroid function. We would suggest therefore that normality of ITI would not be defined as a mean, but as a range within which euthyroidism is maintained.

That beneath a certain critical level of iodine depletion, hypothyroidism occurs, accompanied with modifications of intrathyroidal iodine composition is well documented. On the other hand, not very much is known as to what happens at the other end of the scale when iodine is administrated in excess to normal glands. Apparently "normality" can be maintained to concentration of up to about 1.0 mg/gr tissue of even 1.85 mg/gr (Table 1).

Some hints to this problem have been reported in Japan (19): in the region of Hokkaido, the population subsists on a iodine rich diet and although many of them present with goiter, they are euthyroid and the goiter subsides when iodine is withdrawn. A significant discharge of iodide after perchlorate administration suggested that iodide had been accumulated under inorganic form. Furthermore, an increased MIT/DIT relation was demonstrated after chromatography of thyroid tissue as well as a decrease in $T_3/T_4$ ratio. Excess iodide can thus lead to goiter formation without impairing overall thyroid function. Whether it can also cause hyperthyroidism in normal glands is discussed in another chapter of this monograph.

## 2. 2. Thyroid disease

In normal thyroid glands, iodopolypeptides, iodoproteins and other iodocompounds of uncertain nature exist besides the exchangeable iodine pool (14,09,20), that presumably do not take part in hormonogenesis although it cannot be excluded that iodide derived from their deiodination may reenter the circuit of hormone formation. Some of these compounds are found in blood under the form of non butanol extractable iodine (NBEI), representing what is known as the iodide leak (21). Increased concentration of NBEI is found in various thyroid diseases (21,22) and many different abnormal iodocompounds have been extracted from diseased human glands (21). In these circumstances therefore a great heterogeneity of iodinated substances are assessed by XRF, including some that will not contribute to hormonogenesis.

It ensues that the correlation between ITI and measurements in vivo and the levels of circulating thyroid hormones should be viewed with great caution in thyroid disease.

This chemical heterogeneity is well documented in edemic (23) and simple goiter (15) and the functional and morphological heterogeneity of simple goiter has recently been reviewed by Studer (12). This group has produced evidence that suggest that during the course of growing of the goiter, excessive replication of epithelial cells occurs with subsequent generation of new follicles of widely different structure and function. It results that newly formed follicles, that later may grow into clinically detectable nodules, may present different functional anomalies (defects in iodide trapping, organic binding, thyroglobulin synthesis, exocytosis and for endocytosis) within the same gland. This forms the basis of a likely explanation for the pathogenesis of "hot" and "cold" nodules.

XRF scanning of the thyroid very clearly demonstrates this differentiation in human glands (10). The classical heterogeneity of simple goiter as seen upon scintiscans, already by itself a reflection of the phenomenon, is also found by XRF, but not necessarily with comparable distribution. Some non-toxic hot nodules contain non detectable amounts of stable iodine (Figure 1).

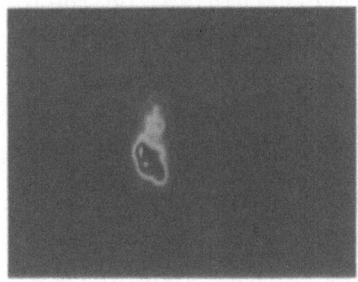 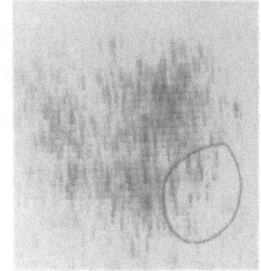

Figure 1. Autonomous nodule with a low ITI conc.
Left : $^{99m}$Tc scan ; Right : XRF scan.

On the other hand, some toxic nodules present with a high amount of ITI (Figure 2) and some do not. The fact that most cancerous lesions of the thyroid contain less iodine has been demonstrated in vivo by XRF (24,25,26).

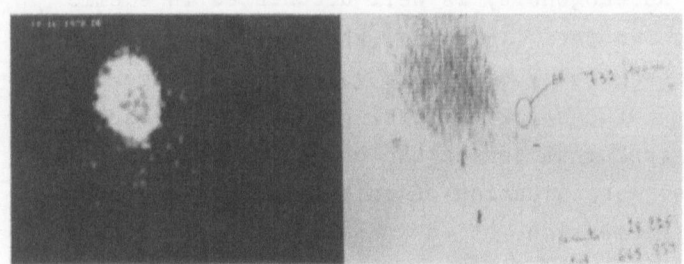

Figure 2. Toxic nodule with high ITI conc.
Left : $^{99m}$Tc scan ; Right : XRF scan.

Nodular goiters respond also differently to iodine treatment. The danger of treating these patients with iodine has been stressed following massive treatment in a goitrous endemic area (27), but also in sporadic goiter (28). We are currently following up goitrous patients treated with small doses of iodine. Although we avoided to include nodular goiters in the trial, some exceptions were seen. Some non-toxic "hot" nodules containing no detectable iodine and having a low TITI showed an increase to normal of their TITI with no concentration in the nodule. Although they remained "hot" on the scintiscan, the patients did not develop hyperthyroidism. Some "cold" nodules with a high iodine content did not evolve either toward hyperthyroidism. On the other hand, the clinical evolution of patients with nodular toxic glands with increased iodine content follow closely the evolution of this TITI.

These examples illustrate the functional heterogeneity of the nodules, but cast no light as to the nature of what one is measuring with XRF. A detailed review of the functional and morphological changes in nodular goiter, as well as its iodocompounds composition has recently been published by

Studer and Romelli (29). It follows also that finding different Iconc in different parts of the gland might not have a direct correlation with the peripheral thyroid function.

Nevertheless it can be assumed from a practical point of view that in the in vivo assessment of ITI in simple goiter, one measures essentially efficient functioning thyroid tissue. Indeed, evidence obtained in our department suggests the existence of critical level of ITI concentration in this disease below which thyroid function decompensates: it was found that serum thyroglobulin concentration starts to rise when ITI concentration reaches about 0.2 mg/gr (30). This figure is keeping with the results obtained in vitro already cited (15): below 0.25 mg/gr tissue, the normal distribution of iodoaminoacids in thyroglobulin is impaired.

The same reasoning holds true for atrophic autoimmune thyroiditis (AAT). NBEI is found increased in the serum of these patients (31) and abnormal iodocompounds are present in these atrophic glands (32), the iodine of which will be measured by XRF. Nevertheless, a significant correlation between TITI and circulating thyroid hormones was found during the continuous evolution of AAT from the euthyroid states up to the moment when basal TSH starts to rise in serum (17,18). As stated above, this breakpoint lies around 2 to 3 mg TITI. Because these glands are atrophic, there is no way to assess their weight in vivo either by palpation, echography or planimetry after XRF scintigraphy. It is however possible to estimate this weight approximatively, making use of the XRF measurements. In our hands the weight of normal glands, estimated by means of planimetry (33), is 25 gr. As we found the mean TITI to be 9 mg, 2 to 3 mg TITI would corresponds to a weight of about 7 gr and the TITI concentration would lie around 0.3 mg/gr. These calculations were made to point out that approximatively the same critical level, under which the thyroid decompensates, is found in AAT as it is in simple goiter.

Other interesting information obtained by means of XRF that allows to show the dissociation of hormonogenesis and storage funtion has been reported in the literature. In Hashimoto's thyroiditis a transient iodide trapping defect could be evidenced (34). In subacute thyroiditis, iodine stores are depleted (35) and it has been shown that uptake of iodine resumes more rapidly than iodine storage in this disease (Chapter IX).

## 2.3. Iatrogenic thyroid disease

With the exception of iodine-containing ones, no drug is known to be the cause of hyperthyroidism. The mechanisms by which some drugs, others than iodine-containing ones, provoke hypothyroidism are relatively well documented (36). In this section, we will briefly discuss dysthyroidism as a result of iodine contamination, stressing the role of XRF measurements in its detection.

Hypothyroidism induced by iodine is well documented and it has been postulated that is is the iodide ion that is responsible, a phenomenon classically known in the Wolff-Chaikoff effect (37). This blocking effect has been shown to be enhanced by antithyroid antibodies (38,39), antipyrine (40) and lithium (41). The pathogenesis of the clinical entity known as "iodide goiter" (37) in which goiter and/or hypothyroidism appears and subsides concomittantly with iodide intake and withdrawal, has been related to the Wolff-Chaikoff effect that had been demonstrated in animal. In our laboratory a few cases of iodide goiters were discovered by means of XRF (see example in Fig. 3). A correlation could be established between the clinical state of the patient and its TITI, demonstrating the validity of the pathogenic hypothesis. Because an important part of iodine can be washed out by perchlorate in these cases, it has been assumed that iodide accumulates under inorganic form (42). On the other hand, evidence has been produced of the existence of an organic iodine pool in which iodine is rapidly accumulated in rats chronically treated with high doses of iodide, and from which iodine , in a form other than iodothyronines, is quickly released (43).

IODINE GOITRE
—————— (CASE REPORT)
DE W... KAREL        58 Y
NOV. 77 :   CHOLECYSTOGRAPHY
JAN. 78 :  - WEIGHTGAIN, SLOWNESS, COLDNESS,
             SLEEPINESS,
           - GOITRE
           - REFLEXOMETRY 300/400 MSEC.

| | JAN. | SEPT. | DEC. |
|---|---|---|---|
| T$_4$ (5 - 11 MIGROG/DL) | 4.8 | 5.9 | 6.6 |
| T$_3$ (74 - 158 NG/DL) | 58 | 123 | - |
| TSH (0 - 7 MIU/ML) | 3.4 | 1.0 | 3.0 |
| TRH | 3.4 17.8 18.2 | - | - |
| ITI (9 MG ± 3.7) | 26.0 | - | 9.5 |

Figure 3 :

Example of a case of iodide goiter.

Whereas the XRF measurement obviously cannot make the difference between these iodocompounds, especially as hypothyroidism can be the result of the administration of complex substance containing iodine, it can be used as an aid in the diagnosis and the treatment of these particular situations.

No non-iodinated compound is known to induce hyperthyroidism and it is assumed that the iodinated ones produce this effect by means of the iodide liberated. It is also generally admitted that hyperthyroidism due to iodide will preferentially set in in already diseased glands (44). It should be stressed that some of these drugs interfere with the peripheral conversion of T$_4$ to T$_3$ (45,46) rendering the diagnosis of hyperthyroidism by the laboratory tests difficult and that at least one, amiodarone, blurrs the clinical signs (47) so that the clinical diagnosis may also be difficult. There is however no reason to believe that the peripheral effects of these drugs can result in dysthyreosis, stressing the role of the liberated iodide itself, either at the periphery or in the thyroid. Reports start to appear that demonstrate by means of XRF the accumulations of iodine in the gland during treatment with various iodine containing drugs (36,47,48,49). Different accumulation and releasing periods have been documented and some correlation between the ITI and the levels of circulating hormones could be shown.

As long as one does not know the rate of accumulation of the drug in the gland, nor its release mechanism and most importantly its deiodination rate, no direct relationship between the measured ITI and thyroid function can be inferred. Nevertheless, although no information as to the nature of what one is measuring by XRF can be gathered, these studies bring into light two aspects of the importance of assessing TITI in these circumstances. For instance, one can conclude from the data published by Haberman et al, (48,49), in keeping with our own experience (50), that when the iodine containing agent has been withdrawn, the urinary iodide excretion reaches normal levels long before the ITI. This means that normal urinary iodide excretion does not exclude iodine contamination. Another aspect will be discussed in Chapter XI in more details: normal glands should accumulate a certain amount of the iodocompound. Dysthyroidism as a consequence of this administration was found to be accompanied with a lower TITI than expected, giving a hint to the presence of an underlying thyroid disease.

3. TREATMENT WITH STABLE IODINE.

Iodine deficiency is a worldwide problem and eradication of cretinism, hypothyroidism and goiter is possible with iodine supplementation on a large scale in overt endemic goiter areas (01). Recent reports demonstrate that, because iodine deficiency is one of the etiological factors of sporadic goiter, treatment of individual cases can be beneficial (Chapter VIII).

The problem is that large doses of iodide are inhibitory and no general argreement exists as to the useful level of replacement therapy. Varying inhibitory doses of plasma iodide have been reported: as low as 0.006 mg/dl (33,51) or higher 0.03 mg/dl (42). This inhibitory effect has been shown to be related to the relative concentration of iodide on both sides of the thyroid cell membrane (37). Empyrical regimens showed that the administration of 0.2 mg KI a day normalized the serum $T_3/T_4$ ratio after 4 weeks (52), that a discontinuous supplementation of 2 mg KI every two weeks resulted in the normalisation of different parameters of thyroid functions as well as in a decrease of goiter size (13). As seen in Chapter VIII, the same beneficial effects, related to the increase in ITI concentration can be achieved with a daily intake of 0.1 to 0.15 mg KI.

Data recently obtained in our laboratory (unpublished) suggest that in normal man even very small doses of iodide can inhibit $T_4$ and $T_3$ secretion and that this inhibition is modulated by the intrathyroidal iodine stores. Ten normal volunteers took in 1 mg iodide (1.309 mg KI) once a week during 6 weeks and 2 mg weekly during another 6 weeks. The results of serum $T_3$, $T_4$, $rT_3$, as well as TITI are shown, under standardized form, in Figure 4. A steady incorporation of iodine is obvious. Serum $T_4$ and $T_3$ concentrations decrease in parallel and increase spontaneously (the regimen of iodide, 1 mg once a week, is maintained) after 3 weeks and the same fluctuation is observed when the dosis iodide in doubled. The hormone levels remain within normal ranges. No statistical fluctuation of $rT_3$ was seen. This demonstrates that 1 or 2 mg iodide, i.e. physiological quantities, do not prevent replenishment of iodine stores in "normal" glands in our area, which is relatively iodine deficient. On the other hand, the physiological doses provoke a temporary inhibition of hormone secretion depending upon the TITI present in the gland. This observation suggests that an inhibitory dosis of iodide will be different in different regions of the world, related to the alimentary iodine intake.

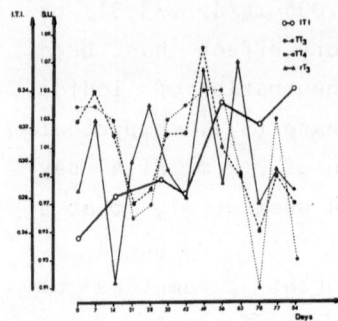

Figure 4 : Variations of $T_4$, $T_3$, $rT_3$ and ITI after administration of 1 mg iodide once a week during 6 weeks and 2 mg a week during another 6 weeks. The results represent the mean in 10 normal subjects, expressed in standardized units.

4. CONCLUSIONS

Iodine is essential for a normal thyroid function. Animal studies, epidemiological studies in man without direct measurement of iodine stores and in vitro studies on thyroid slices have demonstrated the importance of TITI variations in the etiology of some thyroid disorders. Direct assessment of TITI in vivo in man and most importantly its evolution in time is now possible by means of XRF. The major part of stable iodine in the gland represents mainly functional thyroid tissue, with some exceptions, such as in the case of contamination with iodinated drugs or radiological contrasts. An excellent correlation between XRF measurements and iodine content as measured by chemical methods was found by most laboratories and variations of TITI correlating with the clinical state of patients has also been shown. Therefore, if one keeps in mind some restrictions due to methodological problems and other factors, the XRF method can be used for physiopathological and clinical studies in man. It has already confirmed mechanisms that were classically known from indirect evidence and it is hoped that it will extend our knowledge of thyroid function in relation to stable iodine.

## REFERENCES

01. Dunn J.T., Meideiros-Neto (Eds) 1975. Endemic goiter: continuing threats to world health. PAGO, Wahinton, Scientific Punlication Nr 292.
02. Delange F.M., Ermans A.M. 1976. Endemic goiter and cretinism. Naturally occuring goitrogens. Pharmac. Ther.C. 1: 57-93.
03. Grayson R.R. 1960 Factors which influence the radioactive iodine thyroidal uptake test. Am.J.Med., March: 397-415.
04. Aabach H.S.1976. Jodutskilleslse i urin, i relasjon til til forskjellige viktige fodemidler. Intern. Rapport F-365, Forsvarets Forskningsinstitutt. Norwegian Defence Research Establishement, Norway.
05. Hoffer P.B., Jones W.B., Crawford R.B., Gottschalk A. 1968. Fluorescent Thyroid Scanning: a new method of imaging the thyroid. Radiology 90: 342-344.
06. Stanley M.M. 1949. The direct estimation of the rate of thyroid hormone formation in man. The effect of the iodide ion on thyroid iodine utilisation. J.Clin. Endocrinol. & Metab. 9: 941-954.
07. Berson S.A., Yalow R.S. 1954. Quantitative aspects of iodine metabolism. The exchangeable organic iodine pool and the rates of thyroidal secretion, peripheral degradation and fecal excretion of endogeneously synthesized organically bound iodine. J.Clin.Invest. 33: 1533-1552.
08. Koutras D.A., Alexander W.D., McHarden G.R., Sir E. Wayne. 1964. Effect of small iodine supplementation on thyroid function in normal individuals. J.Clin. Endocrinol. 24: 857-862.
09. DeGroot L.J. 1966. Kinetic analysis of iodine metabolism. J.Clin.Endocrinol. 26: 149-173.
10. Jonckheer M.H., Deconinck F. 1982. X-Ray-Fluorescence determination of stable iodine in the thyroid gland. A review. Acta Clinica Belgica 37: 92-102.

11. Jonckheer M.H. 1982. Thyroid Physiology: Hormonogenesis and Iodine Storage. In: Progress in Radiopharmacology 3, P.H. Cox (Ed), Elsevier, North Holland, in press.
12. Studer H. 1982. A fresh look at an old thyroid disease: euthyroid and hyperthyroid nodular goiter.J.Endocrinol. Invest. 5: 57-68.
13. Ermans A.M., Verelst J. 1980. Acute effects of supra-physiological doses of iodine in the human being: management of non-toxic goiter. J.Mol.Med. 4: 199-202.
14. Ermans A.M., Kinthaert J., Delcroix C., Collard J. 1968 Metabolism of Intrathyroidal Iodine in Normal Men. J.Clin.Endocrinol. 28: 169-180.
15. Ermans A.M., Kinthaert J., Camus M. 1968. Defective intrathyroidal iodine metabolism in nontoxic goiter: inadequate iodination of thyroglobulin. J.Clin. Endocrinol. & Metab. 28: 1307-1316.
16. Bigos S.T., Ridgway E.C., Kourides I.A., Maloof F. 1978 Spectrum of pituitary alterations with mild and severe thyroid impairment. J.Clin.Endocrinol & Metab. 46: 317-325.
17. Jonckheer M.H., Vanhaelst L., Deconinck F., Michotte Y. 1981. Atrophic Autoimmune Thyroiditis: relationship between the clinical state and intrathyroidal iodine as measured in vivo in man. J.Clin.Endocrinol. & Metab. 53: 476-479.
18. Jonckheer M.H., Coomans D., Massart D.L., Vanhaelst L., Deconinck F. 1982. The application of SIMCA pattern recognition to the study of autoimmune atrophic thyroiditis. Nucl.Med.Com. 3: 70-77.
19. Suzuki H., Higuchi T., Sawa K. Ohtaki S., Horiuchi Y. 1965. Endemic coast goitre in Hokkaido, Japan. Acta Endocrinol. 50: 161-176.
20. Otten J., Jonckheer M., Dumont J.E. 1971. Thyroid albu-min. II. In vitro synthesis of a thyroid albumin by normal human thyroid tissue. J.Clin.Endocrinol. & Metab. 32: 18-26.
21. DeGroot L.J., Stanbury J.B. 1975. The thyroid and its diseases. John Wiley and Sons, New York.
22. Bastenie P.A., Ermans A.M. (Eds). 1972. Thyroiditis and thyroid function. Pergamon Press, G.B.
23. Ermans A.M. 1978. Disorders of iodine deficiency: ende-mic goiter. In: The Thyroid Gland, Werner and Ingbar (Eds)., Harper & Row, Maryland, Hagerstown: 537-553.
24. Patton J.A., Hollifield J.W., Brill A.B., Lee G.S., Patton D.D. 1976. Differentiation between malignant and benign solitary thyroid nodules by fluorescent scan-ning. J.Nucl.Med. 17: 17-21.
25. LeBlanc A.D., Bell R.L., Johnson P.C. 1973. Measurement of 127-I concentration in thyroid tissue by X-Ray fluorescence. J.Nucl.Med. 14: 816-819.
26. Tadros T.G., Maisey M.N., Ng Tang Fui S.C., Turner P.C. 1981. The iodine concentration in benign and malignant thyroid nodules measured by X-ray fluorescence. Brit.J.Radiol. 54: 626-629.

27. Stewart J.C. 1975. Epidemiology and Pathogenesis of Iodine-Induced Thyrotoxicosis in Northern Tasmania. New Zealand Med.J.81: 25-26.
28. Ermans A.M., Camus M. 1972. Modifications of thyroid function induced by chronic administration of iodide in the presence of "autonomous" thyroid tissue. Acta Endocrinol. 70: 463-475.
29. Studer H., Ramelli F. 1982. Simple Goiter and Its Variants: Euthyroid Hyperthyroid Multinodular Goiters. Endocrinol.Rev. 3: 40-61.
30. Jonckheer M.H., Unger J., Coomans D., Decoster C. 1982. Relationship between serum thyroglobulin and intra-thyroidal stable iodine in euthyroid goitrous patients. In: Progress in Radiopharmacology 3, P.H.Cox (Ed.), Elsevier, North Holland, in press.
31. Bastenie P.A., Ermans A.M. (Eds) 1972. Thyroiditis and Thyroidal Function. Pergamon Press, Oxford.
32. Kivikangas V., Lamberg B.A., Maenpaa J. 1970. Thyroidal iodine and proteins in autoimmune thyroiditis. Scand.J. Clin.Lab.Invest. 25: 263.
33. Mandart G., Erbsman F. 1975. Estimation of thyroid weight by scintigraphy. Int.J.Nucl.Biol. 2: 185-188.
34. Barbato A.L., Bekerman C., Refetoff S. 1977. Transient iodide trapping defect in Hashimoto's thyroiditis detected by the combination of radionuclide and fluorescent scanning. Br.J.Radiol. 50: 827-830.
35. Rappaport B., Block M.B., Hoffer P.B. et al. 1973. Depletion of thyroid iodine during subacute thyroiditis. J.Clin.Endocrinol. & Metab. 36: 610-611.
36. Jonckheer M.H. 1980. Iatrogenic hypothyrodism. In: Bastenie P.A., Bonnijns M., Vanhaelst L. (Eds). Recent progress in diagnosis and treatment of hypothyroid conditions. Excerpta Medica, Congress Series Nr 529, Amsterdam, Ned.: 15-28.
37. Wolff J. 1969. Iodide goiter and the pharmacolic effects of excess iodide. Am.J.Med. 47: 101-124.
38. Braverman L.E., Woeber K.A., Ingbar S.H. 1969. Induction of myxedema by iodide in patients euthyroid after radioiodine or surgical treatment of diffuse toxic goiter. New Engl.J.Med. 15: 816-821.
39. Hall R., Turner-Warwick M., Doniach D. 1966. Autoantibodies in iodide goitre and asthma. Clin.exp.Immunol. 1: 285-296.
40. Begg T.B., Hall R. 1963. Quart.J.Med. 32: 351.
41. Temple R., Berman M., Robbins J., Wolff J. 1972. J.Clin.Invest. 44: 1277.
42. Raben M.S. 1949. The paradoxical effects of thiocyanate and of thyrotropic on the organic binding of iodine by the thyroid in the presence of large amounts of iodide. Endocrinol. 45: 296-304.
43. Nagataki S., Shiwume K., Nakao K. 1966. Effect of chronic graded doses of iodide on thyroid hormone synthesis. Endocrinology 79: 667-674.

44. Vagenakis A.G., Braverman L.E. 1975. Adverse effects of iodide on thyroid function. Med.Clin.North Amer. 59: 1075.
45. Burger A.G., Lambert M., Cullen M. 1981. Interference de substances medicamenteuses dans la conversion de T4 en T3 et rT3 chez l'homme. Annales Endocrinol. (Paris) 42: 461-469.
46. Larsen P.R. 1982. Thyroid-Pituitary Interaction. New Engl.J.Med. 1: 23-32.
47. Jonckheer M.H. 1981. Amiodarone and the Thyroid Gland. A Review. Acta Cardiol. 36: 199-205.
48. Habermann J., Leisner B., Witte A., Pickardt C.R., Scriba P.C. 1982. Iodine contamination as a cause of hyperthyroidism or lack of TSH response to TRH stimulation (Results based on a screening investigation) J.Endocrinol.Invest. 5: 153-156.
49. Habermann J., Leisner B., Pickardt C.R., Witte A., Scriba P.C. 1981. Influence of acute iodine incorporation on thyroid function and thyroidal iodine content. Acta Endocrinol.Suppl. 240: 20.
50. Jonckheer M.H., Deconinck F., Swaenepoel L. 1980. Upon the importance of differentiating between two forms of hyperthyroidism by means of X-ray fluorescence scanning. In: Stockligt J.R., Nagataki S. (Eds). Thyroid Research VIII. Australian Academy of sciences, Canberra, Australia: 637-640.
51. Feinberg W.D., Hoffman D.L., Owen C.A. 1959. The effects of varying amounts of stable iodide on the function of the human thyroid. J.Clin.Endrocinol. & Metab. 19: 567- 582.
52. Reinwein D., Klein E. 1960. Der Einfluss des Anorganischen Blutjodes auf den Jodumsatz der Menschlishen Schilddruse. Acta Endocrinol. 35: 485-494.

VIII ENDEMIC NON-TOXIC GOITER

B. LEISNER

## 1. INTRODUCTION

A non-toxic goiter is defined as an enlargement of the thyroid gland which is not due to thyroiditis or malignancy, maintaining an euthyroid hormone status (41).

The WHO definition of a goiter endemic area is when more than 10% of the population have goiters (14). For many endemic goiter regions the inverse relationship between goiter incidence and daily iodine supply has been clearly established (25). Iodine deficiency is seen to be the main manifestation factor of the non-toxic goiter (14), even though other goitrogens may act additionally under iodine deficiency (24). The iodine content of normal thyroid and goiter tissue has become more interesting since different intrathyroidal iodine compartments are known, among which only the exchangeable pool may be assessed by short term radioiodine studies (4,47,48), and secondly because the reduced iodine concentration of thyroid tissue possibly represents a permissive factor for the proliferative response to TSH (5,8). Up to now the iodine concentration data of thyroid tissue have mostly been derived from the chemical analysis of specimens obtained during surgery or at autopsy (17,28). This provides only a momentary status. Changes in the iodine content due to varying exogenous factors could only be demonstrated in experiments on animals.

Several authors reported the values of total iodine content of goiters using the in-vivo fluorescent scintigraphy introduced by Hoffer et al. (29). Most of these studies were carried out in countries with sufficient nutritional iodine intake (33,49,51). The few published in-vivo measured iodine concentration data were based on the thyroid weight, estimated from the scintigraphic parameters (e.g. plane area, size of the lobes etc.), which has been shown to be very inaccurate(32).

In patients from the goiter endemic area of Southern Germany we determined directly in-vivo the I-127 concentration by means of a modification of the usual fluorescent technique, based on single point measurements independently from the scanning. Moreover, the question was raised whether variable iodine supply affects this parameter in different age-groups and if so, to what extent. Changes of the goiter size were documented objectively using the quite accurate ultrasonic method for thyroid volume determination (31,55).

## 2. PROCEDURE

### 2.1. Fluorescent scintigraphy

We used the fluorescent scanning system ORTEC model 4820 with a concentric source-detector configuration adapted to a PICKER Magna Scanner 500. After completion of the fluorescent scan and according to the individual scintigraphic pattern, several (at least three) measurements of the $K_\alpha$ count rate were made at different points of the thyroid. The counts were corrected for background scattering by an identical registration at an extrathyroidal site of the neck with the same energy window centered on the $K_\alpha$ peak. The very important tissue absorption ("half-value-layer" 12,5 mm) was compensated for using cross-sectional ultrasound scans of the neck at the points of the previous fluorescent measurement (Fig. 1). From the calibration curves obtained with varying concentrations of stable iodine and different phantom thickness (10 - 30 mm), the regional iodine concentration was determined (40,44).

In order to validate the technique, we examined deep frozen human thyroid tissue particles of about 300 mg. They were obtained at autopsy with no selection of patients. The fluorescent analysis was carried out in a plexiglass holder. It was designed to locate the particles exactly and with high reproducibility within the focus of the excitation radiation. Subsequently the iodine concentration was determined chemically after alkaline hydrolysis, using the Sandell-Kolthoff reaction in a TECHNICON autoanalyzer. There was an excellent agreement between the values obtained in both ways ( Fig. 2). However, a slight systematic underestimation by the chemical method was noted, probably due to iodine losses during the several steps of the sample preparation, as demonstrated by Robertson et al. (59) with the neutron activation analysis. Different samples from the same thyroid showed a variation of the iodine concentration of up to 30%, concordingly in both the fluorescent in-vitro and in the chemical analysis. This was stressed by the results of a separate study designed to evaluate the meaning of iodine concentration measurements compared to the total iodine:

In 40 patients we determined the mean iodine concentration as mentioned above. Additionally it was derived from the total iodine content of the gland, divided by the sonographically measured thyroid volume (Fig. 3). There was a good correlation with a coefficient of r = 0,9059, although the maximal error (95% of the cases) was as high as 36%, the mean error being ± 15,2%.

## 2.2. Thyroid volume determination

Patients were examined in the supine position with the neck hyperextended. Using a compound ultrasound scanner equiped with a 5 MHz transducer, transverse scans were made at right angle to the longitudinal body axis. These scans were spaced at 1 cm intervals. A computer program was developed, which calculated the thyroid areas of the sections based upon digitizing of the contour of the gland (Fig. 4). From these areas and the number of sections was computed the thyroid volume (V) according to the formula:

$$V = k \times S \times \sum_{i=1}^{i} F_i$$

where k is a correction factor for photographic reduction, S the section distance and $F_i$ the thyroid area of the scan(31). The digitizing was performed by means of a SUMMAGRAPHICS x/y graphic converter interfaced with a CBM computer. With a section

distance of 1 cm the maximal error was 11,8%, as shown with
pig kidney phantoms (31). Comparing  thyroid cyst volumes calculated by this method and determined by needle aspiration
respectively, the maximal error was 7,8%.

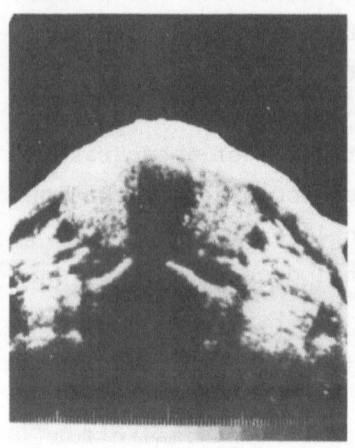
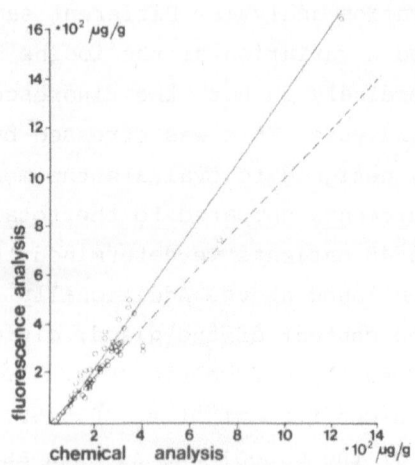

FIGURE 1. Transverse ultrasound scan of a normal thyroid used
for gland thickness measurement.

FIGURE 2. Iodine concentration: chemical analysis plotted against
fluorescent analysis (y = 1,406 x - 20; r = 0,979).

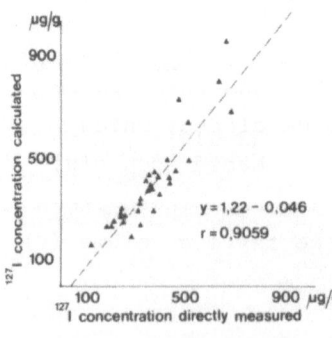
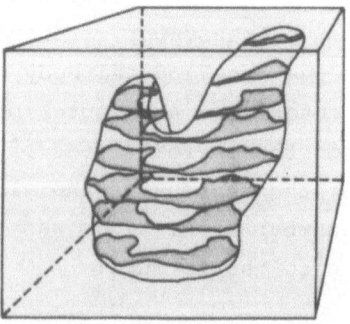

FIGURE 3. Comparison between the results of direct iodine concentration measurement and concentration calculated from the total I-127 content and thyroid volume. Max.error = 36%.

FIGURE 4. Schematic "reconstruction" of the thyroid based on
ultrasound scan planes.

## 3. RESULTS

The iodine concentration (IC) of <u>normal thyroids</u> averaged 370 µg/g. There was no correlation between the IC and the age, the thyroid hormone serum levels and the responsiveness of TSH to TRH (Tab. 1).

TABLE 1. Iodine-127 concentration and thyroid function ( $\bar{x} \pm s_x$ ).

| | n | $^{127}I$ (µg/g) | $T_4$/TBG (µg/mg) | $TSH_{30'}$ (µU/ml) | age |
|---|---|---|---|---|---|
| Normals | 49 | 370 $\pm$ 79 | 3,96 $\pm$1,05 | 8,84 $\pm$2,89 | 25,2 (18-52) |
| Goiter adults | 65 | 288 * $\pm$109 | 3,66 $\pm$0,90 | 8,72 $\pm$5,92 | 38,5 (18-73) |
| Goiter children and adolescents | 77 | 296 * $\pm$112 | 3,57 $\pm$0,71 | 2,47 $\pm$1,15 ($\overline{TSH}_{30'}$) | 13,2 ( 6-17) |

* significantly different from normal value

In <u>non-toxic goiter</u> the average IC was significantly below the normal both in adults and in children. Only juvenile patients showed a weak positive correlation between the $T_4$/TBG ratio and the IC. No relationship was found between goiter volume and IC because even small goiters often contained only minimal iodine amounts. On the contrary the IC of goiter tissue was age-dependent: in the patients over 50 the IC was significantly lower than in the under 40's. TSH responsiveness to TRH was not more accentuated than, and the mean $T_4$/TBG ratio was not beneath that of normals (Tab. 1).

In the following, a longitudinal study under iodide load will be reported. Only patients under 35 years of age were included because of the well known prevalance of autonomous thyroid tissue in longstanding goiters.

- 15 patients with nodular (n=4) and diffuse (n=11) goiter grade II (WHO) received a substitution dose of 150 µg KI daily over 3 - 5 months. The IC did not increase significantly. The

only effect observed was the reduction of the TSH response to
TRH (Tab. 2).

TABLE 2. $^{127}$Iodine concentration of goiters in adults before
and during iodide supplementation (150 µg daily) for 3-5 months.

|  | $^{127}I$ (µg/g) | $T_4$/TBG (µg/mg) | $T_3$ (ng/dl) | $TSH_{30'}$ (µU/ml) |
|---|---|---|---|---|
| Before iodide | 236 $\pm$ 74 | 3,58 $\pm$0,94 | 179 $\pm$ 98 | 8,28 $\pm$5,50 |
| During iodide | 230 $\pm$ 96 | 3,71 $\pm$0,96 | 165 $\pm$111 | 5,14 * $\pm$2,93 |

* significantly different from value before iodide

- 46 children and adolescents (6 - 17 years) were examined before and during 4-8 months of iodide treatment (100 - 150 µg
daily). For comparison a group (n=29) under L-thyroxine therapy (2 µg/kg body weight) was also studied. The results are sum-
arized in Table 3.

TABLE 3. $^{127}$Iodine concentration of goiters in children and
adolescents before and during iodide therapy (100-150 µg daily)
for 4-8 months and before and during L-thyroxine therapy (6 month)

|  | $^{127}I$ (µg/g) | $T_4$/TBG (µg/mg) | $TSH_{0'}$ (µU/ml) |
|---|---|---|---|
| Before iodide | 299 $\pm$134 | 3,69 $\pm$0,74 | 2,32 $\pm$0,91 |
| During iodide | 570 * $\pm$197 | 3,85 $\pm$0,56 | 1,41 * $\pm$0,68 |
| Before L-thyroxine | 305 $\pm$134 | 3,64 $\pm$0,63 | 2,47 $\pm$1,15 |
| During L-thyroxine | 243 # $\pm$144 | 4,15 # $\pm$0,89 | 1,29 # $\pm$1,0 |

*,# significantly different from values before iodide and
L-thyroxine respectively.

During iodide treatment the mean IC increased from 299 µg/g up to 570 µg/g, i.e. by 80%. The $T_4$/TBG ratio remained unchanged, whilst the mean TSH serum level decreased from 2,32 to 1,41 µU/ml (39%). 83% of the patients had TSH levels below 2,1 µU/ml (considered as normal), compared to only 44% before therapy (Tab. 4).

TABLE 4. Normal and elevated TSH serum levels of children with goiter before and during iodide and L-thyroxine treatment.

| | n | TSH normal | TSH elevated |
|---|---|---|---|
| Before iodide | 41 | 18 (44%) | 23 (56%) |
| During iodide | 41 | 34 (83%) | 7 (17%) |
| Before L-thyroxine | 68 | 31 (46%) | 37 (54%) |
| During L-thyroxine | 29 | 25 (86%) | 4 (14%) |

Under L-thyroxine therapy the low IC decreased even further. The $T_4$/TBG ratio slightly increased. The fall in the mean TSH-levels was marginally more noticeable and the fraction of TSH-levels below 2,1 µU/ml virtually equal with 86% (Tab. 4). Along with the TSH decrease, the goiter volume of our juvenile patients diminished significantly, but nevertheless did not reach normal values. According to the rather rough empirical estimation proposed by some pediatricians for individuals below age 20 (i.e. normal thyroid weight (grams) should equal age (years)), we should have found a mean weight of 12,9 g in our patients; in fact it was initially 26,4 g and diminished by 37% to 16,6 g (Fig. 5). Interestingly enough, we did not find a substantially better response of the goiter size to the standard L-thyroxine therapy: the volume decreased by 40% on the average. When comparing thyroid volumes above and below 20 ml, the increase of the IC under iodide was more accentuated in the latter, whereas volume reduction prevailed in the former (Fig. 6). However, shrinkage of the goiter and raise of the iodine concentration were not systematically related: the same degree of IC increase may be paralleled by double volume loss.

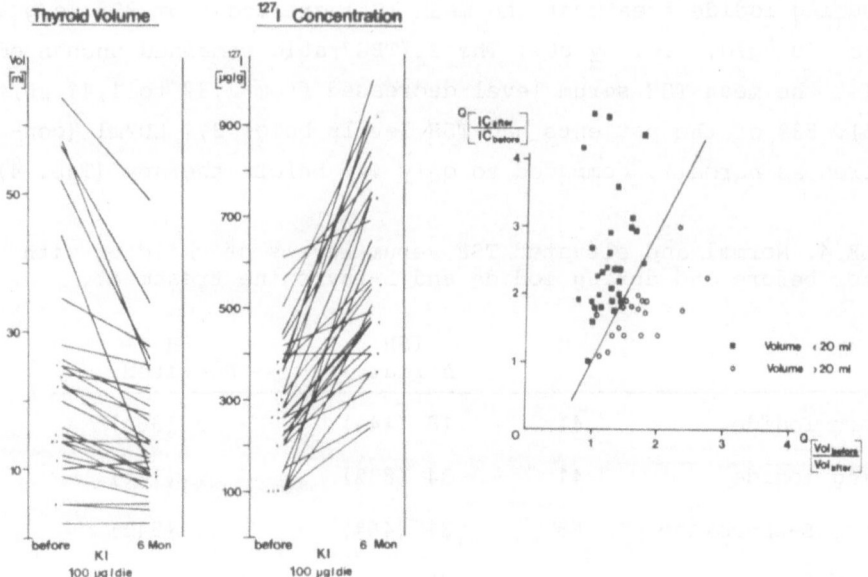

FIGURE 5. Thyroid volume decrease and iodine concentration increase in children and adolescents with non-toxic goiter under iodide treatment.

FIGURE 6. Comparison between the iodine concentration increase and the volume decrease ratios during iodide treatment of juvenile goiter patients (right).

4. DISCUSSION

Several authors reported methods for measuring the iodine content of the thyroid in vivo. Besides the complicated procedures of neutron activation analysis (7) and x-ray spectrophotometry (26,37), the fluorescent technique has been used successfully (2,29,33,39,49,51). The clinical usefulness of such iodine measurements is limited by two factors:

- size differences of the thyroids cannot be taken into account.
- inhomogeneity of the intrathyroidal iodine distribution is neglected.

For a direct comparison with our results the only data available are those of LeBlanc et al.(6) and Tadros et al.(64), which were obtained using XRF in-vitro. Additionally the chemi-

cal values and those calculated from total iodine content can
also be considered as long as normals are concerned. High IC
values are reported from countries with normal to supraoptimal
iodine supplies, the highest being found in regions where the
maximal I-131 uptake is as low as 10-5% under more than 700 µg
iodine intake daily (Tab. 5).

TABLE 5. Thyroidal iodine concentration reported in the literature.

| Author | Country | Year | Technique | n | $^{127}$I (µg/g) |
|---|---|---|---|---|---|
| Agerbaek | Denmark | 1974 | chem. analysis | 217 | 400 |
| Arosenius | Sweden | 1964 | chromatography | 6 | 615 |
| Dimitriadou | UK | 1966 | " | 8 | 550 |
| Ermans | Belgium | 1968 | " | 9 | 620 |
| Fisher | USA | 1969 | " | 8 | 1030 |
| Nagataki | Japan | 1972 | " | 20 | 648 |
| LeBlanc | USA | 1973 | XRF analysis in-vitro | 9 | 980 |
| Larsen | USA | 1975 | immunoassay | 11 | 630 |
| Robertson | USA | 1976 | NAA | 15 | 500 |
| Imamura | Japan | 1979 | XRF analysis in-vivo | 30 | 549 |
| Kohler | Switzerland | 1979 | | | |
| Kohler | Switzerland | 1979 | chem. analysis | 16 | 414 |

In contrast our normal IC of 380 µg/g agreed well with a
maximal radioiodine uptake of 47% and the low mean dietary
iodine of 46 µg daily (25). The lack of correlation between
the IC and the thyroid function parameters is explained by the
more efficient iodine utilization by the normal gland even under
iodine deficiency (43). Normal responsiveness of TSH to TRH
indicates, that an equilibrated hormone status may be maintained
by means of thyroid autoregulation (63).

IC values of goiter tissue ranging below those of the normal
have been reported earlier. A similar tendency is also seen in
the data of LeBlanc et al. (6) and Tadros et al.(64)(sporadic
goiter) and Costa et al.(11) and Hellstern et al.(28). The latter
pointed out, that goiter volumes increased at a higher extent
than the stored iodine, which correlated to the findings in
iodine deficient rats(63). Ermans (15) reported similar results
from the extremely iodine deficient area of Uéle/Zaïre, where

the IC of goiters was 80 µg/g, compared to 620 µg/g of thyroids
from normal Belgians. Total iodine, however, was only slightly
reduced (10,1 mg vs. 12,1 mg). Therefore both the reported increased (46) and decreased (38,49) IC values of goiters cannot
be evaluated on a comparative base, due to lack of informations
about the gland size.

The main biochemical findings which contribute to an explanation of the normal or even increased total iodine content despite
a reduced IC, are the following:

Iodine deficiency results in a low iodination of thyroglobu-
line (3,17,58), which demonstrates abnormal sedimentation (35).
It contains much MIT, less DIT, little $T_4$ and only relatively
more $T_3$ (1,56). This newly formed TG remains at the periphery
of the follicular lumen (60). Its preferential hydrolysis libe-
rates less $T_4$ and $T_3$, but much tyrosines. Their intrathyroidal
deiodination furnishes iodine, which is only insufficiently
reutilized (34). In addition, there are iodine pools with a long
period, that are resistant against proteolysis. They are not
available for thyroid hormone secretion (63). Their fraction
increases, when secretion of iodine compounds is not followed
by a corresponding new synthesis of TG. As in other goiter endemic areas, the $T_4$/TBG ratios were low or normal (12). Their
positive correlation with the IC only in juveniles seems to be
due to a less important fraction of iodine compartments with
slow turnover, known to augment with age (42). This tendency
towards reduction of $T_4$ secretion is counterbalanced by slightly
increased $T_3$ serum levels (30,50), dependent on TSH stimulation
(34,63).

Elevated TSH serum levels or TRH responsiveness were found
in individuals from severely iodine deficient regions (9,10,12).
The same is true for children from such areas (21,23). Under
normal iodine supplementation TSH is reported to remain constant
during growth (18,19,36). The mean concentration ranges from
1,5 µU/ml to 2,2 µU/ml. Surprisingly, in mild iodine deficiency,
75-80% of the goiter patients exhibit normal TSH secretion
(3,13,53). Thus goiters persisting at normal TSH levels are
supposed not to be actually subject to significant growth

stimulation (61).

A possible explanation at least of the persistance of goiters despite TSH levels not exceeding the normal range can be drawn from the experiments carried out on rats by Bray (8), that demonstrated an inhibitory effect of iodine on the goitrogenic response to TSH. These results have been supported by in-vitro inhibition of TSH-mediated adenylate cyclase activity and cyclic AMP (5,54) and of some steps of the intermediary metabolism (34) by iodine.

Our measurements of IC and thyroid volume provide for the first time indications that there is some relationship between exogenously induced changes in IC of the thyroid and the actual TSH secretion rate. When treated with the same physiological doses of iodide (100 - 150 µg daily), both adults and children with non-toxic goiter showed a change of the TSH stimulation, documented in the former by decreased responsiveness to TRH and in the latter by a significant reduction of the basal TSH levels. The striking difference between the two groups was the lack of increase of the IC and of goiter regression in the adult patients.

There are several lines of evidence at least in animals, that following a more efficient iodination of thyroglobulin, the $T_4$ secretion is enhanced, which in turn activates the negative pituitary feedback, thus resulting in lower TSH levels (63). It seems plausible that in the case of a longstanding goiter small amounts of iodide, which lead to normal iodination in only few active follicles, may not suffice to increase the overall thyroidal IC. This is in keeping with the well recognized functional and morphological hetereogeneity of goiters, including a decreased exchangeable iodine pool (20,52) and a great number of "cold" follicles (42). Transformation of a diffuse goiter into a colloidal one, which has been demonstrated in the iodine deficient rat following iodide load as well as ceasing TSH stimulation (63), may account for the goiter resistance against the lowering of TSH stimulation.

On the other hand a small additional supply of iodide might be able to raise the IC of a juvenile goiter, since most of its

follicles participate in the more efficient thyroglobulin iodination. The absence of advanced structural alterations of the
goiter probably permits its volume response to the decreased
TSH levels

A lot of epidemiological data also fit well into the assumption that there is some age dependency of the iodine utilization
by the thyroid. 13 years after the onset of iodized salt pro-
phylaxy in Austria, the incidence of "school" goiter diminished
from 31% to 4%. In contrast, 31,8% of the adult women and 13%
of men still had goiters at this time (62). A similar "dying
out" of non-toxic goiter occurred in Switzerland (22). One has
to admit, however, that only the preventive effect on goiter
development has been ascertained by these studies.

Although comprehensive work from developed countries is still
lacking, our findings of goiter regression following iodide
supplementation support the few published data concerning such
effects. Thus earlier observations of a positive action of
iodine on the congenital goiter have been confirmed by Heidemann
and Stubbe (27), who successfully used 100 - 150 µg potassium
iodide daily. Further evidence of the therapeutic efficacy of
iodine was furnished recently by Ermans and Verelst (16) in
ten adult patients treated with 2 mg of potassium iodide every
15 days. Two years after therapy was started, the mean yield
of goiter regression was 33%. In a controlled study with adults
below age 30, Ridder-Dirks (57) found a more impressive response
of the goiter size on a treatment with 1000 µg of potassium
iodide daily than on a standard therapy with 150 µg of L-thyroxine. Moreover, after withdrawal of any substitution, the relapse rate was higher in the L-thyroxine group than in the
iodide group. This was confirmed by our preliminary results
with 600 µg of potassium iodide daily in a similar age-group,
which exhibited a 40% goiter size decrease together with an
increase of the IC by 70% (45).

One would be led to conclude that raising the thyroidal
iodine concentration by moderate iodide supplies is an essential
factor not only for the prevention of goiter but also for a
physiological treatment, at least in children and young adults.

This is indicated by the decrease of both TSH levels and of the
goiter size following iodine replenishment of the gland. It is
tempting but rather speculative at the time being, to relate
our clinical findings to the experimental ones of Bray (8),
who demonstrated the inhibitory effect of iodine on the goitrogenic response to TSH.

REFERENCES

1.  Abrams G, Larsen P. 1973. Triiodothyronine and thyroxine in
    the serum and thyroid gland of iodine deficiency rats.
    J.Clin.Invest. 52 : 2522.
2.  Aubert B, Fragu P, Di Paola M, Rougier P, Tubiana M. 1981.
    Application of x-ray fluorescence to the study of iodine
    distribution and content in the thyroid. Eur.J.Nucl.Med.
    6 : 407.
3.  Beckers C, Cornette C. 1971. TSH-production rate in non-
    toxic goiter. J.Clin.Endocrinol.Metab. 32 : 852.
4.  Berson S, Yalow R. 1954. Quantitative aspects of iodine
    metabolism. J.Clin.Invest. 33 : 1533.
5.  Berthier C, Lemarchand-Béraud T. 1978. Importance of thyroid
    iodine and cyclic AMP, and TSH concentrations on goiter
    formation in rats. Acta endocrinol. 89 : 567.
6.  LeBlanc A, Bell R, Johnson Ph. 1973. Measurement of $^{127}$I-
    concentration in thyroid tissue by x-ray fluorescence.
    J.Nucl.Med. 14 : 816.
7.  Boddy K, Harden R, Alexander W. 1968. In vivo measurement
    of the intrathyroidal iodine concentration in man by acti-
    vation analysis. J.Clin.Endocrinol.Metab. 28 : 294.
8.  Bray G. 1968. Increased sensitivity of the thyroid in iodine-
    depleted rats to the goitrogenic effects of thyrotropin.
    J.Clin.Invest. 47 : 1640.
9.  Chopra K, Hershman J, Hornabrook R. 1975. Serum thyroid hor-
    mone and thyrotropin levels in subjects from endemic goiter
    regions of New Guinea. J.Clin.Endocrinol.Metab. 40 : 326.
10. Coble Y, Kohler P. 1970. Plasma TSH levels in endemic goiter
    subjects. J.Clin.Endocrinol. 31 : 220.
11. Costa A, Cottino F. 1963. Research on iodine meatbolism in
    endemic goiter in Piedmont. Metabolism 12 : 35.
12. Delange F, Camus M, Ermans A. 1972. Circulating thyroid
    hormones in endemic goiter. J.Clin.Endocrin. 34 : 891.
13. Dige-Petersen H, Hummer L. 1977. Serum thyrotropin concent-
    rations under basal conditions and after stimulation with
    thyrotropin releasing hormone in idiopathic non-toxic goiter.
    J.Clin.Endocrinol.Metab. 44: 1115.
14. Dunn J, Medeiros-Neto G. 1974. Endemic goiter and cretinism:
    continuing threats to the world health. Pan American Health
    Organization WHO. Scientific Publication No 292.
15. Ermans A. 1978. Disorders of iodine deficiency: endemic
    goiter. in: Ingbar SH, Werner SC (eds). The Thyroid.
    4th ed. Hagerstown, Harper and Row.

16. Ermans AM, Verelst J. 1980. Acute effects of supra-physio-
    logical doses of iodide in the human being: management of
    non-toxic goiter. J.Mol.Med. 4:199.
17. Ermans AM, Kinthaert J, Delcroix C, Collard J. 1968.
    Metabolism of intrathyroidal iodine in normal man.
    J.Clin.Endocrinol.Metab. 28:169.
18. Fisher DA, Sack J, Oddie TH, Pekary AE, Hershman JM, Lam RW,
    Parslow ME. 1977. Serum $T_4$, TBG, $T_3$ uptake, $T_3$, reverse $T_3$,
    and TSH concentrations in children 1 to 15 years of age.
    J.Clin.Endocrinol.Metab. 45:191.
19. Foley TP, Owings J, Hayford JH, Blizzard RM. 1972. TSH res-
    ponses to TRH in children. J.Clin.Invest. 51:431.
20. McGarack TH, Seegers U. 1959. Status of the thyroid gland
    after age 50. Metabolism 8:136.
21. Garcia-Bulnes G, Cervantes C, Cerbon MA, Tudon H. 1977.
    Serum thyrotropin, triiodothyronine, and thyroxine levels
    by radioimmunoassay during childhood and adolescence.
    Acta endocrinol. 86:742.
22. Gerber D. 1980. Schilddrüsengewichte und Jodsalzprophylaxe.
    Schweiz.Med.Wschr. 110:2010.
23. Golstein-Golaire J, Delange F. 1971. Serum thyrotropin
    level during growth in man. Europ.J.Clin.Invest. 1:405.
24. Greer MA. 1962. The natural occurrence of goitrogenic
    agents. Rec.Adv.Horm.Res. 18:187.
25. Habermann J, Heinze HG, Horn K, Kantlehner R, Marschner I,
    Neumann J. Alimentärer Jodmangel in der Bundesrepublik.
    Dtsch.med.Wschr. 100:1937.
26. Heedman PA, Jacobson B. 1964. Thyroid iodine determined
    by x-ray spectrophotometry. J.Clin.Endocrin. 24:246.
27. Heidemann P, Stubbe P. 1978. Serum 3,5,3'-triiodothyronine,
    thyroxine, and thyrotropin in hypothyroid infants with
    congenital goiter and the response to iodine. J.Clin.
    Endocrinol.Metab. 47:189.
28. Hellstern P, Keller HE, Weinheimer B, Wesch H. 1978.
    Thyroid iodine concentration and total thyroid iodine
    in normal subjects and in endemic goiter subjects.
    Clin.Endocrinol. 9:351.
29. Hoffer PB, Jones WB, Crawford RB, Beck R, Gottschalk A.
    1968. Fluorescent thyroid scanning: a new method of imaging
    the thyroid. Radiology 90:342.
30. Horn K. 1976. Trijodthyronin ($T_3$): Zur Bestimmung und patho-
    physiologischen Bedeutung. München, Urban u. Schwarzenberg.
31. Igl W, Seiderer M, Fink U, Lissner J. 1980. Quantitative
    Volumenbestimmung der Schilddrüse mit Hilfe der Sonographie.
    Nuc Compact 1:11.
32. Igl W, Lukas P, Leisner B, Fink U, Seiderer M, Pickardt CR.
    1981. Sonographische Volumenbestimmung der Schilddrüse.
    Vergleich mit anderen Methoden. Nuklearmedizin 20:64.
33. Imamura K, Sasaki Y, Sekita N, Someya K, Fuji M. 1979.
    Quantitative in vivo measurement of thyroidal iodine content
    by static x-ray fluorescent technique: some preliminary
    clinical observations. Invest.Radiol. 14:316.
34. Ingbar SH. 1972. Autoregulation of the thyroid. Response
    to iodide excess and depletion. Mayo Clin.Proc. 47:814.

35. Inoue K, Taurog A. 1968. Acute and chronic effects of iodide on thyroid radioiodine metabolism in iodine-deficient rats. Endocrinology 83:279.
36. Jackson D, Vanderschueren-Lodeweyckx M, Grant DB. 1975. Thyrotrophin estimation in diagnosis and treatment of childhood thyroid disorders. Arch.Dis.Childhood 50:522.
37. Jacobson B. 1964. X-ray spectrophotometry in vivo. Am.J.Roentgenol. 91:202.
38. Jonckheer M, Deconinck F. 1979. Dissociation between iodine-storage function and hormone formation, as observed with XRF-scanning of the thyroid. Ann.Endocrin. 40:45A.
39. Jonckheer MH, Vanhaelst L, Deconinck F, Michotte Y. 1981. Atrophic autoimmune thyroiditis: relationship between the clinical state and intrathyroidal iodine as measured in vivo in man. J.Clin.Endocrinol.Metab. 53:476.
40. Kantlehner R, Leisner B, Heinze HG, Lissner J. 1979. Untersuchung des Jodgehalts der Schilddrüse durch Fluoreszenzanregung. Fortschr.Röntgenstr. 130:597.
41. Klein E, Kracht J, Krüskemper HL, Reinwein D, Scriba PC. 1973. Klassifikation der Schilddrüsenkrankheiten. Dtsch.med.Wschr. 98:2249.
42. Kohler H, Studer H. 1981. Biochemische Veränderungen in "warmen" und "kalten" Strumaknoten. Therapiewoche 31:1539.
43. Koutras DA, Alexander WD, Harden RM, Wayne E. 1964. Effect of small iodine supplements on thyroid function in normal individuals. J.Clin.Endocrinol.Metab. 24:857.
44. Leisner B, Kantlehner R, Heinze HG, Lissner J. 1979. Klinische Ergebnisse der Schilddrüsenszintigraphie und Jodbestimmung mit Fluoreszenztechnik. Fortschr.Röntgenstr. 130:694.
45. Leisner B, Pickardt CR, Fink U, zur Nieden J, Igl W. 1982. Bestimmung des Schilddrüsenvolumens mittels kleinrechnerunterstützter Sonogrammauswertung nach verschiedenen Therapiemaßnahmen. in: Nuklearmedizin. HAE Schmidt, H Rösler (eds). Stuttgart-New York, Schattauer, p. 757.
46. Meignan M, Galle P. 1978. Exploration thyroidienne par fluorescence X. Etude réalisée chez 140 malades. Nouv. Presse Med. 7:13.
47. Nagataki S, Ingbar SH. 1963. Demonstration of a second thyroidal iodide pool in rat thyroid glands by double isotope labeling. Endocrinology 73:479.
48. Nodine JH, Channick BJ, Sokhos D, Tassoni SD, Perloff WH. 1957. Measurement of the active iodine stores and daily hormonal output of the intact human thyroid. J.Clin. Endocrin. 17:832.
49. Palmer DW, Deconinck F, Swann SJ, Okerlund M, Kaufman L, Hoffer PB. 1976. Low cost intrathyroidal iodine quantification with a fluorescent scanner. Radiology 119:733.
50. Patel YC, Pharoah POD, Hornabrook RW, Hetzel BS. 1973. Serum triiodothyronine, thyroxine and thyroid-stimulating hormone in endemic goiter: a comparison of goitrous and nongoitrous subjects in New Guinea. J.Clin.Endocrinol.Metab. 37:783.

132

51. Patton JA, Hollifield J, Lee GS, Brill AB. 1974.
    Quantitative scanning of thyroidal iodine pools for assess-
    ment of thyroid disease. J.Nucl.Med. 15:522.
52. Petersen F. 1978. Altersabhängige Änderungen im Regelkreis
    der Schilddrüse. Therapiewoche  :961.
53. Pickardt CR, Erhardt F, Grüner J, Horn K, Scriba PC. 1972.
    Stimulation der TSH-Sekretion durch TSH bei blander Struma:
    Diagnostische Bedeutung und pathophysiologische Folgeer-
    scheinungen. Klin.Wschr. 50:1134.
54. Rapoport B, West MN, Ingbar SH. 1976. On the mechanism of
    inhibition by iodine of the thyroid adenylate cyclase res-
    ponse to thyrotropic hormone. Endocrinology 99:11.
55. Rasmussen SN, Hjorth L. 1974. Determination of thyroid
    volume by ultrasonic scanning. J.Clin.Ultrasound 2:143.
56. Reinwein D, Durrer HA, Meinhold H. 1981. Iodine, thyroxine
    ($T_4$), triiodothyronine($T_3$), 3',3,5'-triiodothyronine($rT_3$),
    3,3'-diiodothyronine($T_2$) in normal human thyroids. Effect
    of excessive iodine exposure. Horm.Metab.Res. 13:456.
57. Ridder-Dirks A. 1979. Vergleichende Untersuchungen zur
    medikamentösen Therapie der euthyreoten Struma.
    Thesis Göttingen.
58. Riek M, Kohler H, König MP, Bürgi H, Studer H. 1974.
    Zur Pathogenese des Knotenkropfes. Therapiewoche 24:2332.
59. Robertson I, Boddy K, Hooper MJ, Stevenson RD, McGhie T,
    Alexander WD, Wilson GM. 1976. Total thyroidal content of
    iodine in thyrotoxic patients measured by in-vivo neutron
    activation analysis. Clin. Endocrin. 5:151.
60. Schneider PB. 1964. Thyroidal iodine heterogeneity: "last
    come, first served" system of iodine turnover.
    Endocrinology 74:973.
61. Scriba PC, Pickardt CR. 1980. Die blande Struma. In: Die
    Krankheiten der Schilddrüse. K Oberdisse, E Klein, D Reinwein
    (eds) 2nd ed. Stuttgart-New York , G.Thieme  p. 493.
62. Steiner H, Zimmermann G. 1978. Die Epidemiologie der ende-
    mischen Struma unter Jodsalzprophylaxe. Wien.med.Wschr. 4:476.
63. Studer H, Kohler H, Bürgi H. 1974. Iodine deficiency. In:
    Endocrinology vol.III: Thyroid. MA Greer, DH Solomon (eds)
    Washington DC, Am.Physiol. Soc.
64. Tadros TG, Maisey MN, Tang Fui SC, Turner PC. 1981. The io-
    dine concentration in benign and malignant thyroid nodules
    measured by x-ray fluorescence. Brit.J.Radiol. 54:626

This work was supported by the Deutsche Forschungsgemeinschaft.

The cooperation of Prof. C.R.Pickardt,M.D., and R.Kantlehner,Ph.D.
and the technical assistance of Mrs. L.Segnitz and Mrs. H.Colling
are gratefully acknowledged.

# IX FEASIBILITY OF IN VIVO XRF DYNAMIC STUDY OF THE THYROID FOLLOWING STABLE IODINE ADMINISTRATION

P. PAVONI, L. RAGANELLA, S. DI LUZIO, G. IZZO, A. MAGRINI

## 1. INTRODUCTION

There are some problems regarding the pratical use of XRF technique in the study of the thyroid as it is performed at present. The first is related to the cost/usefulness ratio.

An X-ray fluorescence scanner is at least as expensive as an analogous piece of equipment for the classical scintigraphy complete with all the necessary accessories. The latter is therefore suitable for use in all field in which "in vivo" nuclear medicine diagnostics are valuable. An X-ray fluorescence scanner developed and built for thyroid investigations may be used to obtain morpho-functional images only of the thyroid; besides, these images show a not better resolution than that of radionuclides images.

This observation concerns the imaging of the thyroid. When we pass from qualitative-semi-quantitative to purely quantitative evaluations there appears to be general agreement regarding the complete overlap of total iodine content values obtained with X-ray fluorescence in normal thyroids and those with various pathological conditions.

This result was to be expected. It should not be forgotten, in fact, that the function of an organ is represented by a succession of dynamic events each of which, when statically "photographed", may not appear to be different in organs with enterely different dynamic behaviour: a photograph of one part of a river may show the same quantity of water indipendently of the speed of the current.

The advantages of morphofunctional studies of the thyroid with X-ray fluorescence with respect to evaluations of a quantitative nature as they are currently performed with the same method, are that on the image we have a spatial comparison, qualitative or semi-quantitative, between areas of the same organ which show a different functional behaviour, i. e., in different dynamic phases at the time of scanning. Patton et al. (3) and Maisey and Tang Fui (2) were thus able to distinguish, in fact, thyroid nodules with malignant characteristics from benign nodules.

An analogous quantitative comparison between different normal and pathological individuals can only be performed on a temporal plane, i. e., comparing the dynamic variations in iodine concentration in the thyroid, in patients given an identical dose of stable iodine.

## 2. MATERIALS AND METHODS

A low cost, static XRF device was used, equipped with a Kr-gas proportional counter and with widely collimated $^{241}$Am sources (2 x 45 mCi or 4 x 15 mCi). A description of the system, background subtraction procedure and characteristic performances have been reported elsewhere (1,4,5).

The minimum detectable limit in the entire thyroid is about 1 mg of iodine.

The radiation dose absorbed by the gland is about 1 mrem for each measurement.

Three normal volunteers were studied.

Following a basal measurement, about .08 mg of iodine (Lugol solution) per Kg body weight were administered orally. Several measurements were then performed during subsequent hours (days), placing the measuring head over the neck in a pre-established position. Time variations in intrathyroidal iodine content were thus assessed in terms of changes in the net counting rate due to the iodine fluorescence X-rays.

## 3. RESULTS

An XRF dynamic study has been performed by our group in a preliminary investigation aimed at assessing the feasibility of this type of study using a low cost XRF device (4). In Figure 1 the results obtained in one normal volunteer after administration of 6.2 mg iodine (.08 mg I/kg body weight) are shown.

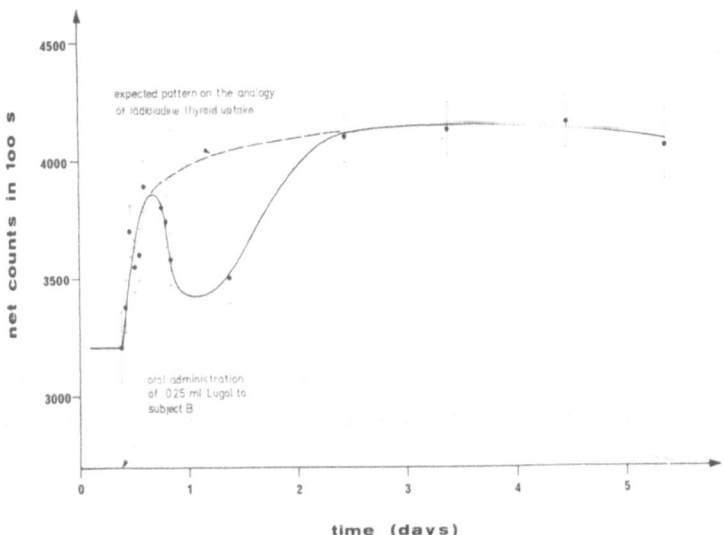

FIGURE 1. Thyroid uptake curve in a normal volunteer after administration of .25 ml Lugol (6,2 mg iodine) (reproduced by permission from ref. (4)).

Successive administrations of increasing quantities of stable iodine to the same subject enabled further slight increases of intrathyroidal iodine to be detected (Fig. 2).

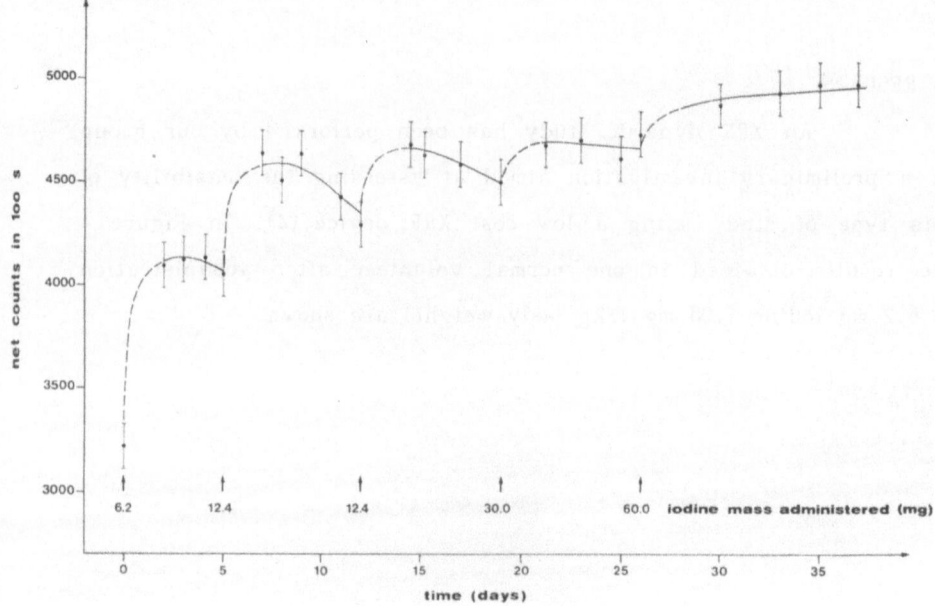

FIGURE 2. Thyroid uptake curve corresponding to periodic administration of increasing quantities of Lugol solution (reproduced by permission from ref. (4)).

The slope of the line expressing the progressive reduction of these increases in thyroid iodine content is shown in Figure 3.

The experiment has recently been repeated, after a few year-interval, in the same subject. The results were very similar to those previously obtained (Fig. 4).

The discharge phenomenon occurring after the 5th hour was confirmed in two other normal subjects (Figg. 5 & 6). However an earlier rise of the uptake occurred in the youngest subject, with respect to the other two subjects (Fig. 6). The experiment was performed in another normal subject with the administration of 100 mg I, but no significant variations in total iodine content of the gland was found within the first 24 hours.

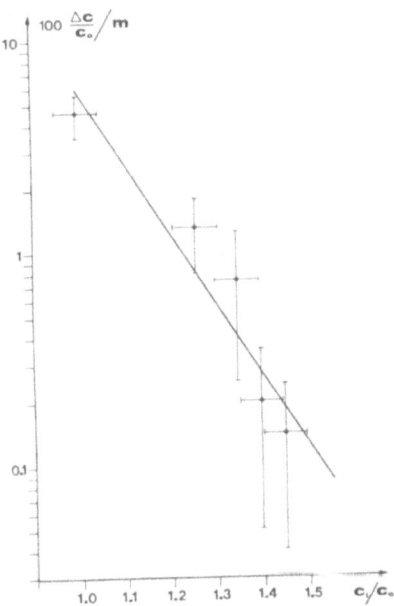

FIGURE 3. Percent variation of intrathyroidal iodine content, per mg of iodine administered, with respect to the quantity of iodine present in the thyroid prior to administration (reproduced by permission from ref. (4)).

This result compares well with the drastic drop in thyroid uptake at 100 mg iodine level, as demonstrated by radio-iodine uptake studies following stable iodine administration, as performed by Sternthal et al. (6).

## 4. DISCUSSION AND CONCLUSION

A schematic representation of the temporal course of the thyroid stable iodine content as observed by us in the normal volunteers is shown in Figure 7. Parameters possibly useful in the evaluation of thyroid function are also shown in the figure.

138

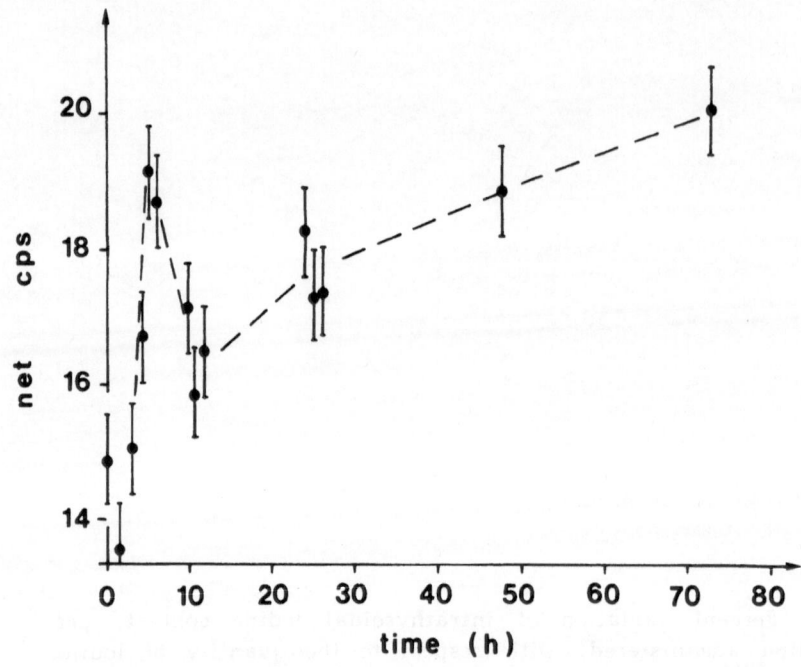

FIGURE 4. Result of the dynamic study in the same subject of figure 1, after about 5 years (age 54). The same quantity of iodine was administered in this istance. Differences in the net counting rates, with respect to figure 1, are due to the lower activity of the [241]Am sources employed in this case and to the different shape of the collimators. Each point represents the mean of 3 independent measurements lasting 300 s each. The statistical error is reported (reproduced by permission from ref. (1)).

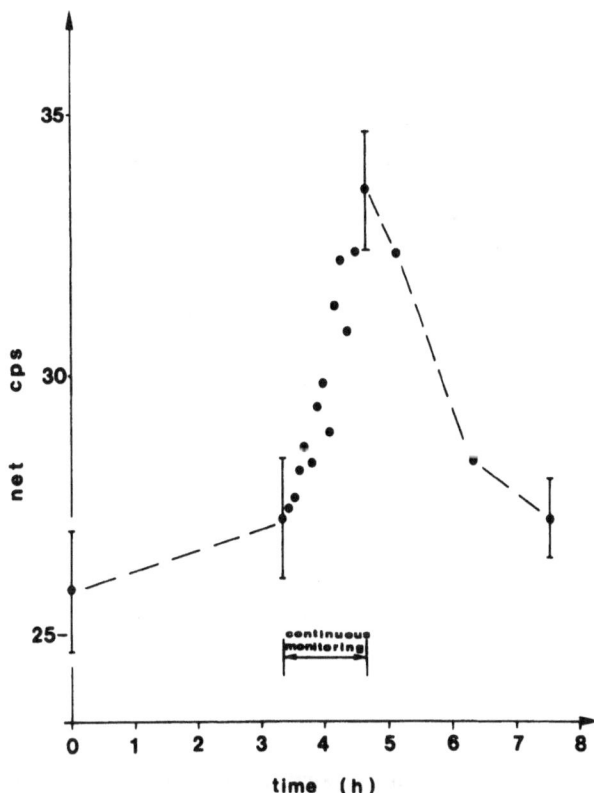

FIGURE 5. XRF dynamic study in a normal volunteer (age 41) after oral administration of .08 mg I/kg body weight. Thyroidal iodine content was continuosly monitored for more than 1 hour with the subject kept in the same position. Counting time was 300 s (reproduced by permission from ref. (1)).

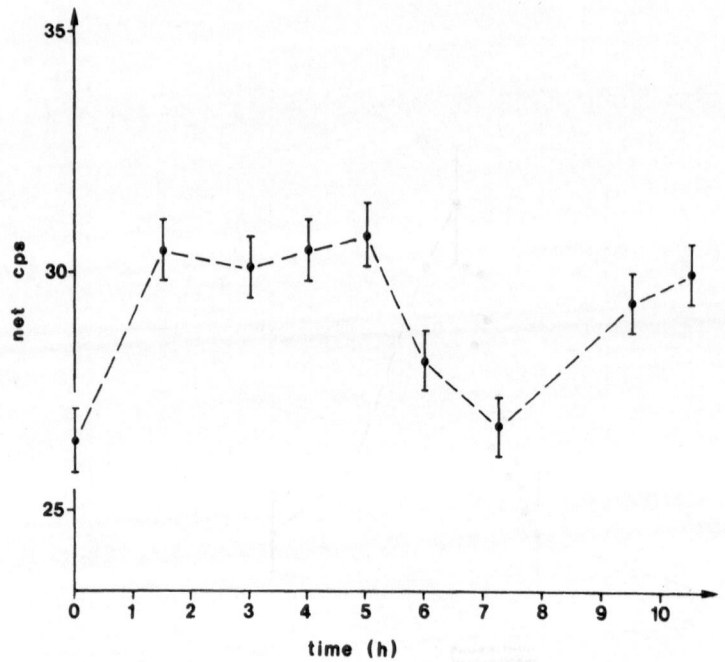

FIGURE 6. XRF dynamic study in a normal volunteer (age 27) after oral administration of .08 mg I/kg body weight. Each point represent the mean of 3 measurements lasting 300 s each. Statistical errors are reported (reproduced by permission from ref. (1)).

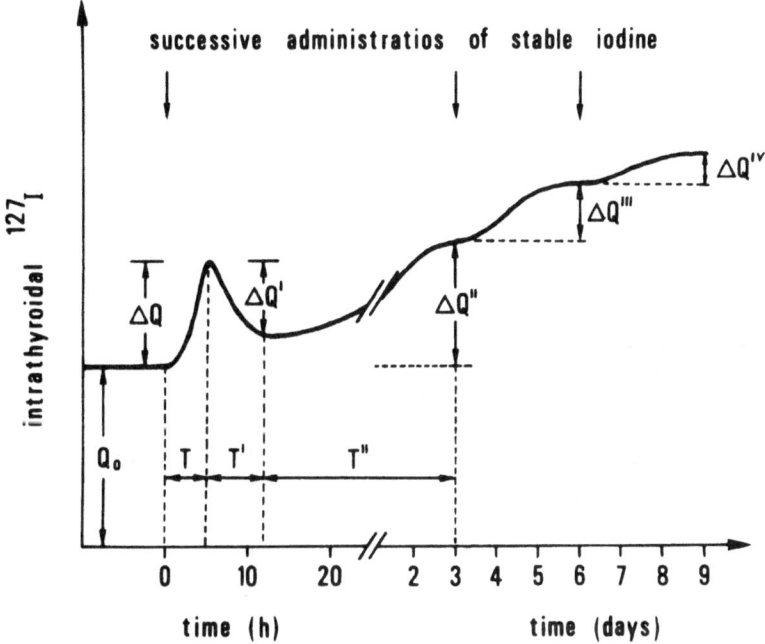

FIGURE 7. Schematic representation of the qualitative course of stable iodine content in the thyroid of a normal subject following intake of .08 mg/kg body weight of stable iodine in fasting conditions. The time course of the thyroidal iodine content following successive administrations of iodine is also shown. The main parameters characterizing the curve are indicated, amongst which those useful for diagnostic purposes may eventually be established. $Q_o$= natural iodine content present in thyroid prior to test. N.B.: this behaviour could, in principle, be studied separately for each thyroid lobe (reproduced by permission from ref. (5)).

142

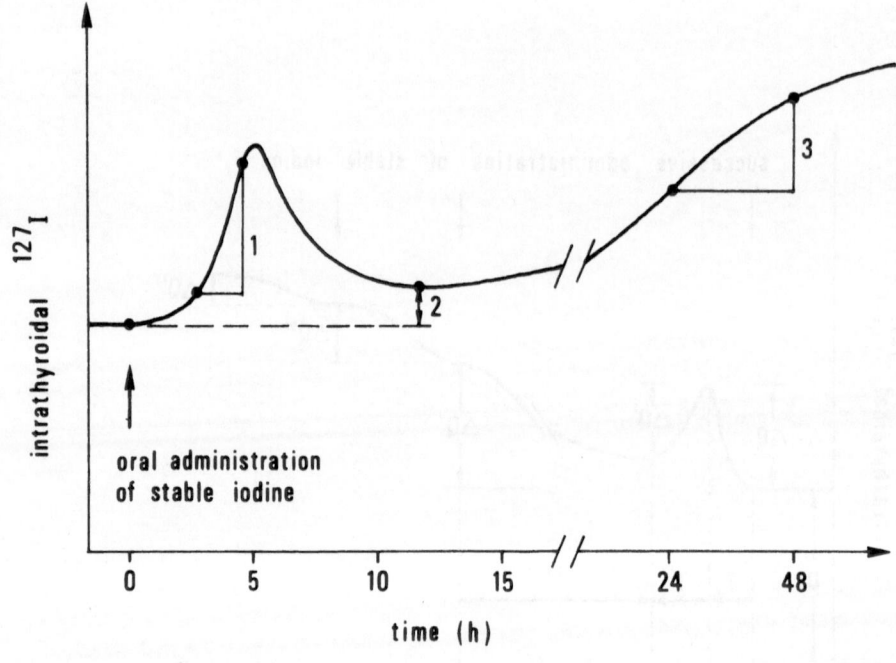

FIGURE 8. Parameters for the evaluation of thyroid function possibly useful for routine diagnostic purposes (see text) (reproduced by permission from ref. (5)).

Determination of some of the parameters shown in Figure 7 may not be feasible since measurements during the 48 hours after administration of the single dose of stable iodine would be necessary. It is worthwhile stressing, at this point, that the dose of .08 mg I/kg body weight appears to be critical: administration of smaller quantities of iodine does not lead to a detectable variation in the thyroid iodine content, whereas we have observed, in agreement with Sternthal et al. (6), that larger quantities markedly inhibit the iodine uptake capacity of the thyroid, thus also reducing the variation in the intrathyroidal iodine content.

Figure 8 shows the parameters for the evaluation of the

thyroid function which will in our opinion be most useful for clinical purposes and the least time-consuming:

1. the mean rising slope of the first part of the curve: this may be obtained with only two measurements (plus a basal measurement) performed within the first 4 hours;

2. the entity of the Wolff-Chaikoff effect (which is well demonstrated using our XRF fluorescence technique under iodine load), measured at about the 10th hour;

3. the mean rising slope of the last part of the curve, measured after the 24th hour with two determinations.

We do not know, at present, whether all of these parameters should always be evaluated to differentiate the pathological forms, since the XRF dynamic study has so far been performed only in normal subjects.

From a technical point of view, the XRF dynamic study is based on the measurement of variations in intrathyroidal iodine content, i. e., on relative measurements. Thus, it offers the advantage of being independent of size, shape and location of the thyroid, although problems occur regarding reproducibility of the measuring position over the neck.

REFERENCES

1. Magrini A., Di Luzio S., Izzo G., Raganella L. 1982. Intrathyroidal iodine determination by X-ray fluorescence. In: X-ray fluorescence (XRF & PIXE) in Medicine, R. Cesareo Ed., Field Educational Italia, Rome, p. 87.
2. Maisey M.N., Ng Tang Fui S.C. 1982. The differentiation between benign and malignant thyroid nodule using X-ray fluorescence with a stationary single detector. Proc. WFNMB Third World Congr., Paris.
3. Patton J.A., Hollifield J.W., Brill A.B., Lee G.S., Patton D.D. 1976. Differentiation between malignant and benign solitary thyroid nodules by fluorescent scanning. J. Nucl. Med. 1:17.
4. Pavoni P., Frazzoli F.V., Magrini A. 1976. Radioisotope X-ray fluorescence technique in the dynamic study of thyroid behaviour under iodine load. Eur. J. Nucl. Med. 1:117.

144

5. Pavoni P. 1982. X-ray fluorescence in physiopathological studies of the thyroid. In: X-ray fluorescence (XRF & PIXE) in Medicine, R. Cesareo Ed., Field Educational Italia, Rome, p. 75.
6. Sternthal E., Lipworth L., Stanley B., Abreau C., Fang S., Braverman L.E. 1980. Suppression of thyroid radioiodine uptake by various doses of stable iodine. N. Engl. J. Med. 303:1083.

X THYROID IODINE CONTENT MEASUREMENT HELPS FOR THE DIAGNOSIS OF HYPER-
THYROIDISM WITH UNDETECTABLE RADIOIODINE UPTAKE

P. FRAGU, M. SCHLUMBERGER, B. AUBERT AND M. TUBIANA

## 1. INTRODUCTION

Fluorescence excitation has already become the method of choice
for thyroid imaging during pregnancy and lactation, in pediatric patients capable of cooperating during the imaging study, and in a large
number of patients undergoing thyroid imaging studies after administration of iodide as contrast media or medicinal (1-3). For the last 6
years, X-ray fluorescence systems have been developed for both imaging
and quantitation of stable iodine within the thyroid gland (2,4-8). The
information derived is related to iodide storage, and clinically useful
data have been obtained in various thyroid disorders (2,4-7,9-13).

The aim of this paper is to report on thyroid iodine content during subacute thyroiditis and hyperthyroidism due to iodine overload.
X-ray fluorescence appears 1°/ to be a differential diagnostic tool
between this two diseases in which radioiodine uptake is undetectable
2°/ an useful tool in the follow-up of the patients during the course
of both diseases.

## 2. METHOD OF MEASUREMENT OF THYROID IODINE CONTENT

The method for the measurement of thyroid iodine content has been
described previously (8). The apparatus consists of an X-ray fluorescence unit (80 kV X-ray excitation beam plus Si (Li) semiconductor)
mounted on the arm of a scanner. The detector axis is vertical and at a
24° angle with the axis of the X-ray beam.

Scintigraphic data are digitized in a Informatek Simis 3 data-
processing unit, which performs acquisition and visualization of the

images on a color TV monitor (Fig. 1). For an iodine line source in a diffusion medium, the spatial resolution varies from 3.2 to 4.1 mm which is better than the resolution of both mechanical scanners and gamma-cameras (3). However, the stable iodine content of large nodular goiters (Fig. 1D) is frequently irregular in distribution (14) and the ability to identify and localize small nodules is much less satisfactory than gamma camera imaging after intravenous injection of $Tc^{99}m$ pertechnetate.

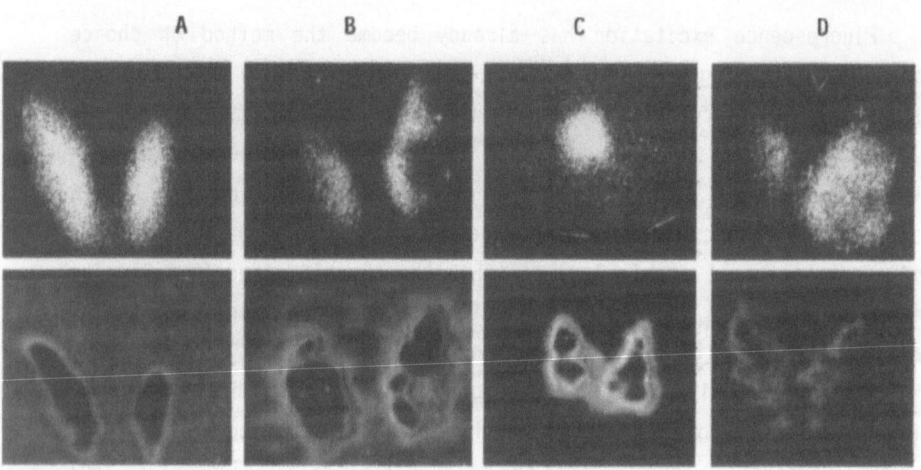

Figure 1 : Comparison $^{99m}Tc$ scan (top) and X-ray fluorescence scan (botton)
A. normal thyroid
B. cold nodule
C. demonstration of suppressed tissue in toxic adenoma.
D. Multinodular goiter. The turnover of iodine of the left lobe is higher than that of the right lobe.

Determination of intrathyroidal iodine content is obtained from a calibration curve established on assays performed with a thyroid phantom (Fig. 2A) and validated by comparing the results obtained with those of chemical analysis of surgery specimens (Fig. 2B). A 2 channels detection method is used. The first channel is set to detect the Kα ray of iodine (28.5 keV) and the background noise in this zone due to the diffusion of X-ray beam in the tissues. The second analyzer detects only those photons that accurately reflect background in the window of

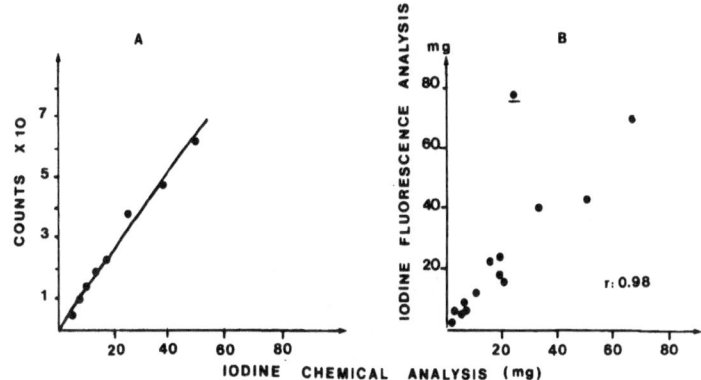

Figure 2 : A calibration curve   B correlation vivo-vitro. ≜ This patient
was not included to compute the linear regression curve.

the first analyzer. This technique leads to the formation  of 2 images in
the data processing unit : one the distribution of iodine and background,
and the other representing only background. After substraction, only the
distribution of iodine in the thyroid is visualized. Reproductibility is $\pm$
5 % and content as low as 1 mg can be accurately evaluated. Furthermore,
this method allows the quantitation of iodine in each lobe and even in
individual nodules (8).


3. THYROID IODINE CONTENT AND THYROID STATE

Figure  3  summarizes  the  iodine  contents  found  in  euthyroid,
hyperthyroid or hypothyroid patients with our system. In the control
euthyroid patients without goiter, the iodine contents  ranged from 2.5 to
27 mg,  which are  in  agreement  with  values  reported  by  other  groups
(Table 1), although the mean value (14.6 $\pm$ 5 mg) is slightly higher.
Furthermore, if we consider that the thyroid weight averages between 20-

Table 1 : Normal thyroid iodine content measured by X-ray fluorescence (mg)

| REPORTS | | MEAN | RANGE | NUMBER OF PATIENTS |
|---|---|---|---|---|
| Patton et al. (1976)(4) | | 10.7 | 2.5 - 22.5 | 30 |
| Thrall et al. (1978)(5) | | 10.1 | 2.4 - 18 | 30 |
| Imamura et al. (1979)(10) | F | 10.6 | 1.6 - 30 | 16 |
| | M | 17.6 | 7.8 - 34 | 14 |
| Okerlund (1979)(2) | F | 9.2 | 4.1 - 19 | 26 |
| | M | 9.9 | 3.8 - 17.5 | 41 |
| Meignan (1979)(6) | | 5 | 1 - 11 | 26 |
| Rougier (1981)(11) | | 15.6 | 8 - 27 | 18 |
| Jonckheer (1981)(12) | | 9 | 1.6 - 16.4 | 48 |

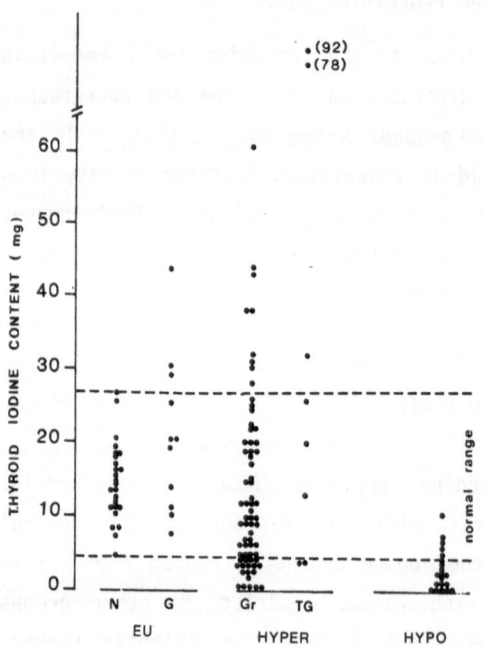

Figure 3 : Thyroid iodine content in euthyroid (Eu) hyperthyroid (Hyper) and hypothyroid (Hypo) subjects. These results confirm and extend the previous report of our group (11)
N : control (26 patients)
G : goiter (11 patients)
Gr : Graves' disease (49 patients)
TG : Toxic goiter (8 patients).

30 g! in normal subjects, our estimated iodine concentration (0.450-0.750 µg/g of tissue) compares very well with the normal range quoted in the litterature for France (15). As reported by Okerlund (2), a significant increase of the total iodine content (21 ± 10 mg) was found in patients with sporadic diffuse goiter, although the iodine per gram of tissue is decreased since the thyroids are characteristically unlarged. This is in agreement with previous findings of our group (16, 17)

In untreated thyrotoxic patients, the range of the thyroid iodine contents (16.5 ± 19.5 mg) is wide in agreement with other studies (2,5,10). 58 % of the patients had an iodine content within the normal range. According to the litterature (18) 90 % of patients with Graves' disease have an increase of their thyroid weight and the iodine concentration of the tissue is consequently decreased in agreement with previous biochemical studies (19) or neutron activation analysis (20). However 20 % of the patients exhibited a value above the upper limit of the normal range, which could not be explained by the increase of the thyroid weight. On the other hand, 22 % of patients had an iodine content below the lower limit of the normal range. This suggest that various types of disorders of thyroid iodine content regulation may be present in hyperthyroidism (21).

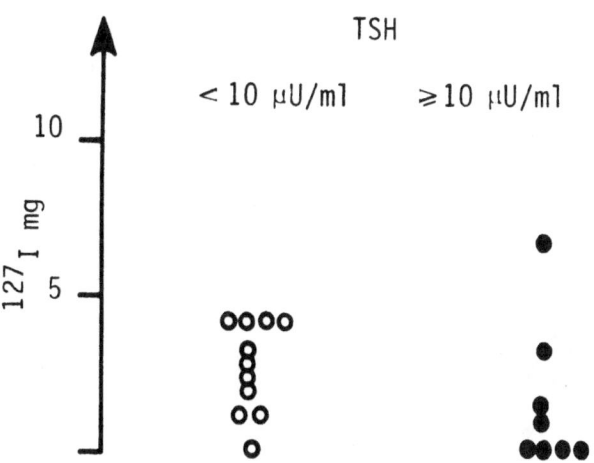

Figure 4 : Iodine content in Hashimoto' disease.

Iodine contents were decreased in hypothyroidism ($3 \pm 3$ mg) and even be undetectable in several patients. In a large proportion of patients with Hashimoto' thyroiditis the iodine contents were undetectable even in the absence of elevated TSH levels (Fig. 4) confirming the strong tendency for these patient to have a low iodine content (1,2,12).

## 4. IODINE STORES IN SUBACUTE THYROIDITIS

Relatively few data were available on the evolution of thyroid $^{127}$I stores in subacute thyroiditis. Several authors have reported normal (5,10) or decreased iodine contents (1,5) during the hyperthyroid phase of the disease. Rapoport et al. (22) observed in one patient, in whom the iodine content was evaluated qualitatively, an early loss of hormone stores and subsequently a low recovery. We report quantitavive data on thyroid iodine contents obtained in 12 patients throughout the course of subacute thyroiditis developed on previously normal thyroid gland (8 cases) or on

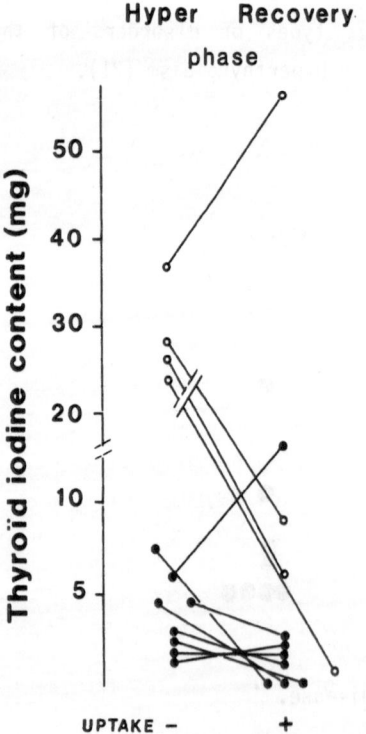

Figure 5 : Time course changes in thyroid iodine content during the early phases of subacute thyroiditis developed in a normal thyroid (●——●) or goitrous gland (○——○)

goitrous gland (4 cases). Part of these results have been reported previously (13).

During the initial hyperthyroid phase of the disease, no patient exhibited detectable $^{99m}$Tc or $^{123}$I uptake and the iodine stores were not completely depleted (fig. 5). When thyroiditis had developed in a normal thyroid, the iodine content (4.5 $\pm$ 2 mg) was about 3 times lower than normal values ; in patients with goiter it was elevated but was still within the normal range of euthyroid goitrous patients. There was no correlation between the iodine content of the gland and circulating thyroid iodine hormone levels $(T_4+T_3)$.

During the early recovery phase of the disease, the radioactive uptake of the thyroid was measurable, and thyroid scans show a homogenous distribution of the tracer in all the patients. The iodine content of the gland increased only in 3 patients (from +35 to + 105 % over the initial values respectively) (Table 2). However in one of these 3 patients, the iodine content decreased again from 13.5 to 6 mg 17.5 months after the end of therapy. In the other patients, iodine contents decreased (from - 32 % to - 100 % of the initial value) even when the disease was developed on a previous goitrous gland. Nearly complete iodine depletion was observed in 4 patients. No correlation was found between the decreases in the thyroid iodine content (expressed as a percent of the initial values) observed during this phase and circulating thyroid iodine hormone levels $(T_4 + T_3)$ observed during the hyperthyroid phase of the disease. Furthermore, the degree of iodine depletion did not seem to be related to the severity of the disease, since patients, in whom a severe depletion was observed, were able to maintain a euthyroid state (Table 2).

Time course changes in thyroid iodine content may be different in the two lobes (Fig. 6) generally one lobe was already depleted at the time of diagnosis while the other lobe subsequently lost its iodine.

Following complete remission, a slow and progressive restoration of iodine stores was observed (Fig. 6 and 7). The thyroid iodine content started to increase only after the elevation of serum TSH and when thyroid blood levels remained stable within the euthyroid range. This increase was slow and the iodine content remained low for 1 year after complete remission (Table 3) although the patients were clinically and biologically euthyroid.

Table 2 : Subacute thyroiditis : biological data at recovery phase

| CASE | $T_3$ ng/dl | $T_4$ µg/dl | TSH µU/ml | THYROID $^{127}$I mg | %a |
|---|---|---|---|---|---|
| Normal gland | | | | | |
| 1 | 150 | 6.6 | 6 | 13.4 | +109 |
| 2 | 127 | 6.5 | 4 | 2.4 | - 51 |
| 4 | 180 | 6.4 | 6.8 | 0 | -100 |
| 5 | 117 | 6.8 | 5.5 | 1.1 | - 68 |
| 7 | 81 | 3.3 | 7.5 | 0. | -100 |
| 8 | 120 | 4.6 | 5 | 0.6 | - 56 |
| 14 | 80 | 2.3 | 7.6 | 1.7 | - 32 |
| 15 | 109 | 8.5 | 9.9 | 2.2 | + 35 |
| Goitrous gland | | | | | |
| 11 | 96 | 6 | 7.5 | 53 | + 45 |
| 12 | 131 | 8.7 | 2.5 | 6 | - 75 |
| 13 | 96 | 4.7 | 4.8 | 9 | - 68 |
| 16 | 85 | 4.2 | 6 | 0.8 | - 100 |

a increase or decrease over the initial value

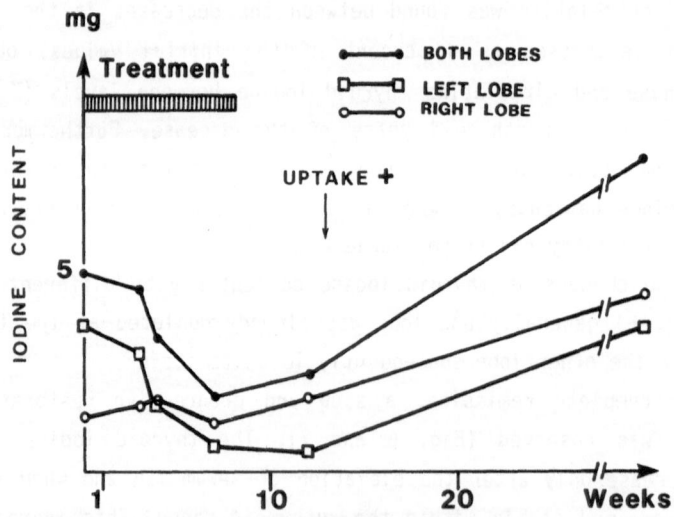

Figure 6 : Changes in the iodine content of each lobe during a subacute thyroiditis. In this special case, changes in iodine content in each lobe mirrored the clinical symptoms : depletion took place as pain and tenderness appeared first in one and then in the other lobe.

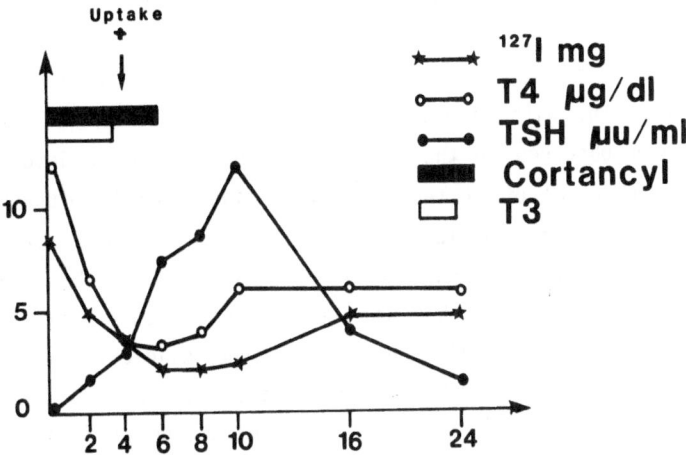

Figure 7 : Time course changes in serum $T_4$, TSH level and thyroid iodine content in one patient with subacute thyroiditis. The arrow indicates a normal thyroid scan.


Table 3 : Late phase of subacute thyroiditis

| Case N° | $T_4$ µg/dl | $TSH_0$ µU/ml | $TSH_{20}$ a | Thyroid $^{127}I$ mg | Time between Remission and Assay (months) |
|---|---|---|---|---|---|
| 1 | 8.2 | | | 6.4 | 17.5 |
| 5 | 8.4 | 2.8 | 21.3 | 5.5 | 13 |
| 6 | 7.4 | 5 | 19 | 7.3 | 12 |
| 8 | 6 | 6.9 | 17 | 4.5 | 15.5 |
| 9 | 4.7 | 4.8 | | 6.4 | 17 |
| 12 | 9.2 | 1.5 | 12 | 9.2 | 18 |
| 14 | 6.9 | 2.6 | | 0 | 9 |
| 16 | 6.8 | 2.1 | | 5.2 | 10 |

a 20 min after TRH injection (200 µg)

It was of interest to know if iodine administration could facili-
tate the restoration of thyroid iodine stores. Iodide solution (KI :
500 µg/day) was administered during 2 to 7 months in 2 control patients

154

and in 5 patients who had previously developed a subacute thyroiditis.
Figure 8 illustrates the time course changes in thyroid iodine content
in two patients choosen as a typical example (one patient with subacute
thyroiditis, one control patient). During iodine treatment a clear
increase of the iodine content (100 % increase over the initial value
before the treatment with KI for both patients) was observed but no
modification was observed in the circulating thyroid iodine level ($T_4$
+ $T_3$). After withdrawal of KI therapy, the iodine content returned to
the initial value in the patient with subacute thyroiditis while it
remained elevated during a much larger time interval in the control
patient. These data suggest that the course of subacute thyroiditis
might be longer than it would appear from the clinical data, the
hormonal assays and the radioiodine thyroid uptake data.

From a practical standpoint, serial determinations of iodine content may be helpful in the differential diagnosis between Graves'
disease and painless thyroiditis (23). In Graves' disease, no change in
iodine content is observed without treatment while in painless thyroiditis a decrease of the iodine content is observed.

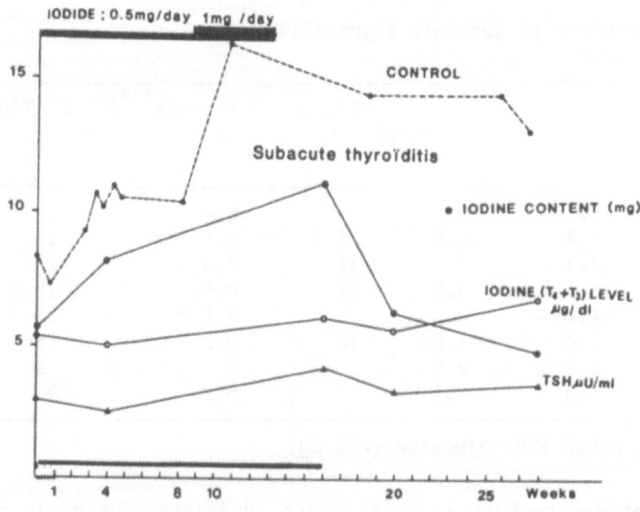

Figure 8 : Effect of iodide administration (500 µg/day) on the iodine
content in a control subject and in a patient of subacute thyroiditis.

## 5. IODINE STORES IN IODINE OVERLOAD

The prime factor controlling thyroid function is thyrotrophin (TSH). Nevertheless, variations in the amount of iodine in the diet may also affect thyroid function and may influence the developpement and the course of thyroid diseases (24-28). Chronic ingestion of iodide or iodide-generating organic compound above the daily requirement for hormone biosynthesis leads to iodide goiter in certain subjects (29) or hyperthyroidism in other patients, particulary in aera of endemic goiter submitted to iodide supplement (29, 30). Iodine induced thyrotoxicosis has been described in patient with previous abnormal gland (goiter, hot nodule, subclinical Graves' disease) (31-33) and iodide unmasked latent hyperthyroidism as shown in figure 9. Iodine induced thyrotoxicosis may also occur on apparently normal thyroid gland (34).

In view of its high iodine content (38 % of iodine by weight) amiodarone, a largely used antiarythmic and antianginal drug, plays a

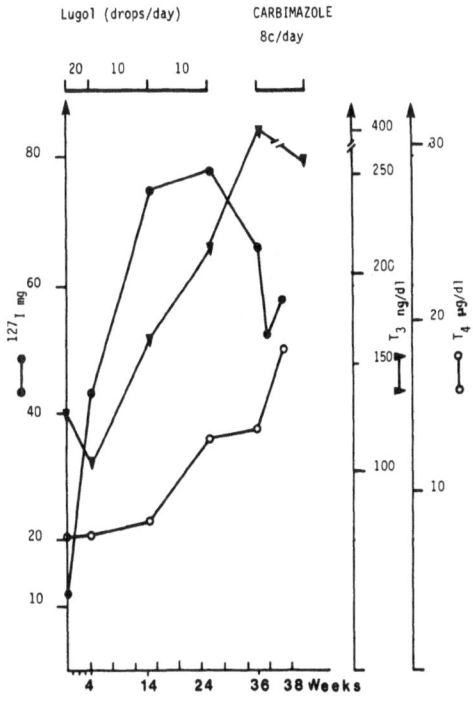

Figure 9 : Time course changes in thyroid iodine content, thyroid hormone blood level in a patient with subclinical Graves' disease treated by lugol solution. A Jod Basedow developed in this patient ; this course illustrates the interest of X-ray fluorescence technique in the follow-up of patient under iodide treatment.

156

particular role and is responsable for most of the iodine induced thyrotoxicosis (35, 36). In order to understand the pathophysiological process of this disease, thyroid iodine content was measured by X-ray fluorescence in 27 patients under amiodarone treatment (fig. 10). 10 patients were euthyroid, 17 hyperthyroid ; in all cases there was no detectable thyroid uptake. These results extend the preliminary report of Leger and al (37).

In patients who remained euthyroid, the mean value of the iodine content (27 $\pm$ 13 mg) was only slighly higher than the upper limit of the normal range and 50 % of the values were in the normal range (fig. 10). This suggest that through an autoregulatory decrease of iodide transport, the intrathyroid iodide concentration remains at a level that permits normal organic binding and hormonal synthesis. In the amiodarone treated patients who had developed hyperthyroidism, the thyroid iodine content was 1.5 fold more elevated (41 $\pm$ 17 mg) than in patients whose remained euthyroid and out of them only 18 % had a normal thyroid content. Whathever was the mechanism by which iodine thyrotoxicosis was induced (amiodarone, lymphography), the changes in thyroid hormones blood levels were parallel to the changes of thyroid

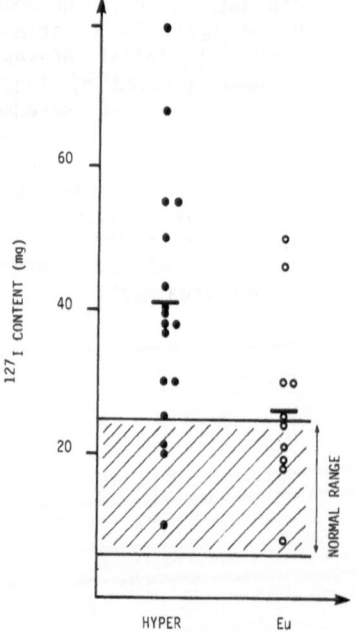

Figure 10 : Effect of Amiodarone treatment on the thyroid iodine content in 27 patients.

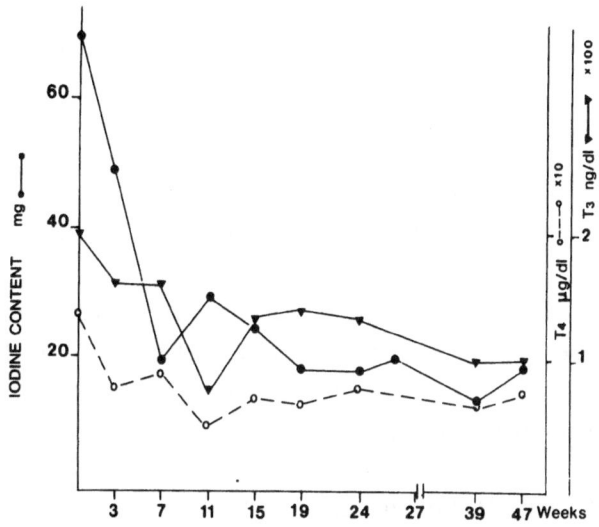

Figure 11 : Spontaneous cure of a case of iodine induced thyrotoxicosis (after lymphography). Times courses changes in thyroid iodine content and thyroid hormone blood levels.

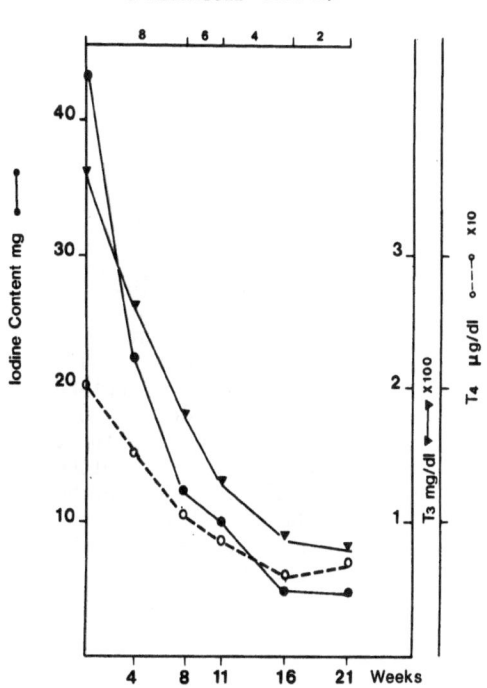

Figure 12 : Time course change in a case of amiodarone induced thyrotoxicosis treated by Carbimazole.

158

iodine content. They returned within the normal range either
spontaneously (figure 11) or after antithyroid drug administration
(figure 12).

All these data support the hypothesis that iodine induced thyrotoxicosis is the consequence of 1) inflated thyroid content 2) absence
of impairment of organic binding and hormonal synthesis despite the
increased iodine content.

From a practical standpoint, the measurement of iodine content is
of interest in hyperthyroid patients without radioactive uptake. A
value above 30 mg, excludes a subacute thyroiditis and suggests an
iodine induced thyrotoxicosis (Fig. 13).

6. THYROID IODINE CONTENT IN THYROTOXICOSIS FACTITIA

Surreptitious ingestion of thyroid hormones may be responsible
for thyrotoxicosis factitia which may be confused with other types of
thyrotoxicosis associated with low radioiodine uptake. Short term

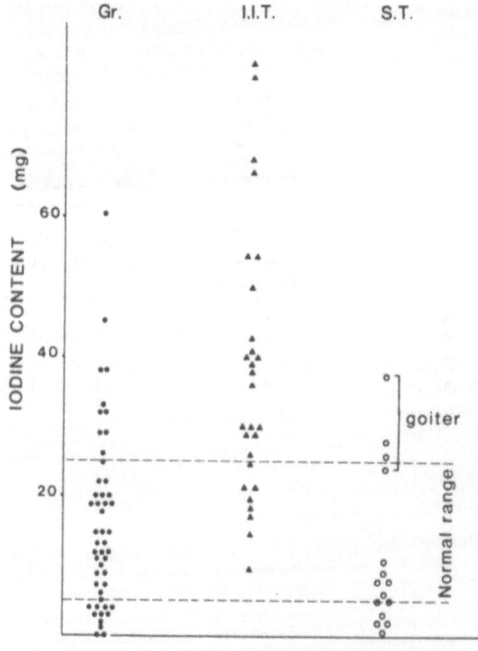

Figure 13 : Interest
of measurement of
iodine content in
hyperthyroidism with
radioactive uptake
(GR : 49 Grave' di-
seases) or without
radioactive uptake
(I.I.T. : 28 iodine
induced thyrotoxico-
sis : S.T. : 15 sub-
acute thyroiditis)

thyroid suppression does not seem to exert a significant effect on the iodine content of the gland (1) but long term treatment decreases it significantly. Serum thyroglobulin (Tg) determination appears to be a complementary tool for the diagnostic evaluation of these patients (36) : serum Tg value is undetectable or in the normal range while it is generally increased in subacute thyroiditis (40).

## 7 - CONCLUSIONS

X-ray fluorescence appears to be a useful tool in the diagnosis of thyroid diseases and opens new field of investigations in thyroid physiopathology. Providing informations about iodide storage, X-ray fluorescence scan is complementary to radioiodine scan which explores the rapid turnover pool of iodine. The developpment of new methods which allows the simultaneous examination of thyroid gland by these both methods (41) may lead to new informations in thyroid pathology. Quantitation of thyroid iodine contents has been also found to be very useful in the diagnosis of thyroid disorders as for instance for hyperthyroid patient without radioiodine uptake. Furthermore with this method it is now possible to study in vivo the autoregulation of the thyroid response to iodide excess in man. Work is in progress in our laboratory to understand the physiopathology of iodine overload.

## REFERENCES

1. Hoffer PB, Bernstein J, Gottschalk A. 1971. Fluorescent techniques in thyroid imaging. Sem Nucl Med 1, 379-389.

2. Okerlund MD. 1979. The clinical utility of fluorescent scanning of the thyroid. In : "Medical Applications of fluorescent excitation analysis". Kaufman L, Price D.C. edt., CRC Press Inc. (Florida) pp 149-160.

3. Fragu P. 1982. Thyroid exploration by imaging techniques including fluorescent scanning. In : "Thyroid Diseases" Beckers C. edt, Pergamon (Paris) pp 89-106.

4. Patton JA, Hollifield JW, Brill AB, Lee GS, Patton DD. 1976. Differentiation between malignant and benign solitary thyroid nodules by fluorescent scanning . J Nucl Med 17, 17-21.

5. Thrall JH, Gillen MT, Johnson MC, Corcoran RJ, Wartofsky L. 1978. Quantitative thyroid fluorescent scanning : Technique and clinical experience. Am J Roentgenol 130, 517-522.

6. Meignan M, Galle P. 1978. Exploration thyroïdienne par fluorescence X. Etude réalisée chez 140 malades. Nouv. Presse Med 7, 13-19.

7. Leisner B, Kantlehner R, Heinze HG, Lissner J. 1979. Klinische Ergebnisse der Schildedrüsenszintigraphie und Jodbestimmung mit fluoreszengtechnik. Fortschr. Röngenstr. 130, 694-695.

8. Aubert B, Fragu P, Di Paola M, Rougier P, Tubiana M. 1981. Application of X-ray fluorescence to the study of iodine distribution and content in the thyroid. Eur. J Nucl Med, 6, 407-410.

9. Pavoni P, Frazzoli FV, Magrini A. 1976. Radioisotope X-ray fluorescence technique in the dynamic study of thyroid behaviour under iodine load. Eur J Nucl Med 1, 117-122.

10. Imamura K, Sasaki Y, Sekita N, Someya K, Fujii M. 1979. Quantitative in vivo measurement of thyroidal iodine content by static X-ray fluorescent technique : Some preliminary clinical observations. Invest Radiol 14, 316-322.

11. Rougier P, Fragu P, Aubert B, Parmentier C, Tubiana M. 1981. Mesure du contenu en iode stable intrathyroidien par fluorescence X. Intérêt et Applications. Path. Biol. 29, 31-37.

12. Jonckheer MH, Vanhaelst L, Deconinck F, Michotte Y. 1981. Atrophic autoimmune thyroiditis : Relationship between the clincial state and intrathyroidal iodine as measured in vivo in man. J Clin Endocr Metab 53, 476-479.

13. Fragu P, Rougier P, Schlumberger M, Tubiana M. 1982. Evolution of thyroid [127]I stores measured by X-ray fluorescence in subacute thyroiditis. J Clin Endocrinol Metab 54, 162-166.

14. Studer H, Ramelli F. 1982. Simple goiter and its variants : Euthyroid and hyperthyroid multinodular goiters. Endocrine Reviews 3, 40-61.

15. Fragu P, Nataf BM. 1977. Human thyroid peroxidase in benign and malign thyroid disorders. J Clin Endocrinol Metab 45, 1089-1096.

16. Tubiana M. 1962. Le goître conception moderne. Rev Franç Etudes Clin et Biol 7, 469-476.

17. Tubiana M, Thomas-Morvan C, Nataf B. 1973. Concentration intrathyroidienne et hormonosynthèse dans divers types d'affections thyroïdiennes. Ann Endocrinol (Paris) 34, 563-577.

18. Mornex R, Orgiazzi JJ. 1980. Hyperthyroidism. In : "The Thyroid gland". De Visscher M edt., Raven Press (New York) pp 279-362.

19. Larsen PR. 1975. Thyroidal triiodothyronine and thyroxine in Graves' desease : correlation with presurgical treatment, thyroid status, and iodine content J Clin Endocrinol Metab 41, 1098-1104.

20. Robertson I, Boddy K, Hooper MJ, Stevenson RD, McGHie T, Alexander WD, Wilson GM. 1976. Total thyroidal content of iodine in thyrotoxic patients measured by in vivo neutron activation analysis Clin. Endocrinol (Oxf) 5, 151-157.

21. Ingbar SH. 1972. Autoregulation of the thyroid. Response to iodide excess and depletion. In "Graves' Disease - 1972". Mayo Clinic Proceedings Forscher B edt, pp 814-823.

22. Rapoport B, Block MB, Hoffer PB, DeGroot LJ. 1973. Depletion of thyroid iodine during subacute thyroiditis. J Clin Endocrinol Metab 36, 610-611.

23. Woolf PD. 1978. Painless thyroiditis as a cause of hyperthyroidism. Subacute or chronic lymphocytic. Arch Intern Med 138, 26-27.

24. Volpe R, Johnston MW. 1962. The effect of small doses of stable iodine in patients with hyperthyroidism. Ann Intern Med 56, 577-589.

25. Braverman LE, Ingbar SH. 1963. Changes in thyroidal function during adaptation to large dose of iodide. J Clin Invest 42, 1216-1232.

26. Williams ED, Doniach I, Bjarnason O, Michie W. 1977. Thyroid cancer in an iodide rich area. A Histopathological study. Cancer 39, 215-222.

27. Ermans AM. 1979. Endemic goiter and endemic cretinism. In : "Endocrinology" DeGroot LJ et al. Edt. Grune et Stratton (New York) pp 501-508.

28. Emrich D, Karkavitsas N, Facarro U, Schürnbrand P, Schreivogel I, Schicha H, Dirks H. 1982. Influence of increasing intake on thyroid function in euthyroid and hyperthyroid states. J Clin Endocrinol Metab 54, 1236-1241.

29. Wolff J. 1969. Iodide goiter and the pharmacologic effects of excess iodide. Am J Med 47, 101-124.

30. Vidor GI, Stewart JC, Wall JR, Wangel A, Hetzel BS. 1973. Pathogenesis of iodine-induced thyrotoxicosis : studies in northern Tasmania. J Clin Endocrinl Metab 37, 901-909.

31. Vagenakis AG, Wang C, Burger A, Maloof F, Braverman LE, Ingbar SM. 1972. Iodine-induced thyrotoxicosis in Boston. N Engl J Med 287, 523-527

32. Sobrinho LG, Limbert ES, Santos MA. 1977. Thyroxine toxicosis in patients with iodine induced thyrotocosis. J Am Endocrinol Metab 45, 25-29.

33. Adams DD, Kennedy TH, Stewart JC, Utiger RD, Vidor GI. 1975. Hyperthyroidism in Tasmania following iodide supplementation : Measurements of thyroid stimulating antibodies and thyrotropin. J Clin Endocrinol Metab 41, 221-228.

34. Savoie JC, Massin JP, Thomopoulos P, Leger F. 1975. Iodine-induced thyrotoxicosis in apparently normal thyroid glands. J Clin Endocrinol Metab 41, 685-691.

35. Jonckheer MH, Blockx P, Kawers R and Wyffels W. 1973. Hyperthyroidism as a possible complication of treatment of ischemic heart disease with amiodarone. Acta Cardiol (Bruxelles) 28, 192-200.

36. Jonckheer MH. 1981. Amiodarone and the thyroid gland. A review Acta Cardiol (Bruxelles) 36, 199-205.

37. Leger AF, Fragu P, Rougier P, Laurent MF, Tubiana M, Savoie JC. 1982. Fluorescent scanning of the thyroid in amiodarone induced thyrotoxicosis. J Nucl Med (submitted for publication).

38. Jonckeer MH, Deconninck F. 1982. X-ray fluorescence determination of stable iodine in the thyroid gland. A review. Acta Clin Belg 37, 92-102.

39. Mariotti S, Martino E, Cupini C, Lari R, Giani C, Baschieri L, Pinchera A. 1982. Low serum thyroglulin as a clue to the diagnosis of thyrotoxicosis factitia. New Engl J Med 307, 410-412.

40. Izumi M, Larsen PR. 1978. Correlation of sequential changes in serum thyroglobulin, triiodothyronine and thyroxine in patients with Graves' disease and subacute thyroiditis. Metabolism, 27, 449-460.

41. Patton JA, Brill AB. 1978. Simultaneous Emission and fluorescent scanning of the thyroid. J Nucl Med 19, 464-469.

XI CLINICAL USEFULNESS OF X-RAY FLUORESCENCE THYROID IODINE
QUANTITATION AND SCANNING.

M.H.JONCKHEER and H.W.WAHNER

## 1. INTRODUCTION

With the use of X-ray fluorescence (XRF) techniques and
under optimal technical and laboratory conditions it is
possible :
1) to quantitate total thyroidal iodine (total organic
and inorganic iodine pool),
2) to quantitate regional thyroidal iodine with the
restriction that a true tomographic evaluation of a given
volume such as a thyroid nodule is difficult and that slices
through the entire thickness of the thyroid gland are being
evaluated and
3) to evaluate relative distribution of iodine in the
thyroid gland by imaging techniques.

The method presently available for clinical studies does
not allow any distinction between inorganic and organic
iodine in the thyroid gland and because of the effect of
overlying tissue on the specific iodine Kα X-ray (half value
layer equals 2 cm of tissue) thyroid tissue not located
immediately under the skin (thyroid cancer metastasis)
cannot be evaluated. The results of iodine measurements with
XRF are expressed in units of weight (mg) of iodine
contained in the area scanned. Additional efforts have to be
extended if a volume measurement is desired. Then, the units
would be mg iodine per volume. The problems concerning the
accuracy of the method are discussed elsewhere in this
monograph.

A critical evaluation of the clinical or research application of XRF in thyroid medicine should center around the question of whether knowledge of a given patient's total or regional iodine content or concentration can significantly aid in the diagnostic decision making process, in the definition of prognosis or therapy or whether it is helpful for investigating specific abnormalities in thyroid diseases.

Presently our diagnostic approach to thyroid disease is based upon 1) recognition of thyroid function mainly by biochemical tests and
             2) evaluation of thyroid morphology by palpation of the neck, biopsy or indirectly by thyroid scanning with radioactive iodide or technetium. In the latter technique, the uptake function ($^{99m}$Tc) or thyroid hormone synthesis function ($^{131}$I) are being used to indirectly demonstrate functioning thyroid follicular tissue as contrasted to hyperfunctioning tissue or to non-functioning abnormal thyroid tissues (malignant or benign). The question then arises of whether the additional information of total or regional iodine content or concentration can be of help in the standard approach of thyroid diagnosis based on function and morphology, as whether this technique opens up new diagnosticly useful criteria.

2. TOTAL IODINE CONTENT OF THE THYROID GLAND

Almost all iodine in the thyroid gland is stored in organic form and present in the colloid of the follicle. The iodine content and concentration in thyroid glands from various populations and goiter regions is given in Table 1. Other examples are shown in Table 1 of Chapter VII. Total iodine content of the thyroid gland is regulated by a complex mechanism. The dietary intake of iodine (extrinsic

Table 1. Thyroid iodine stores and iodine environment.

| Country | Type | Thyroid gland | | Urinary excretion µg per day | Reference |
|---------|------|---------------|--|------------------------------|-----------|
| | | Qg* (mg) | $^{127}I$ concentration (mg per gm) | | |
| | Normal | | | | |
| Belgium | | 12.1 | .62 | 59 | (1, 2) |
| Colombia | | 17.5 | .70 | 229 | (3) |
| Sweden | | 12.9(+) | - | - | (4) |
| United States | | 9.4 | - | 221 | (5) |
| | | 6.3-14.7 | - | 80-225 | (6) |
| | Sporadic goiter | | | | |
| Belgium | | 22.0 | .17 | - | (2) |
| Sweden | | 20.9(+) | - | - | (4) |
| United States | | 4.7-55.6 | - | 31-262 | (6) |
| | Endemic goiter | | | | |
| Chile | | 12.2 | - | 33 | (7) |
| Colombia | (tr) | 15.3 | .29* | 360 | (3)* |
| Congo | (ST) (FT) (tr) | 8.6-15.8 1.9 6.8-36.4 | .08 .16 | 27 41 | (8, 9) |
| Mendoza (Argentina) | | 0.3-12.6 | - | 23 | (10) |
| Misiones (Argentina) | (ST) (FT) | 9.4 4.7 | - - | - - | (11) (11) |

Notes:
  Qg*: Exchangeable organic iodine determined by kinetic methods.
  +: Estimation by spectrophotometric of Heedman et al. (4)
  tr: Iodine prophylaxis or pretreatment with iodine.
  ST and FT: "slow" and "fast" turnover rates of the exchangeable
     organic iodine pool of the thyroid.
  *: Personal communication.

## REFERENCES

(1) Ermans, A.M. and M. Camus. Research concerning the influence of acute exposure to cold on the thyroid function. Aerospace Medical Division, Fort Wainwright, Alaska, Report AAL, TR. 66-7, 1966.
(2) Ermans, A.M., J. Kinthaert, and M. Camus. J. Clin. Endocrinol. 28: 169, 1968.
(3) Wahner, H.W., E. Gaitan, and P. Correa. J. Clin. Endocrinol. 26: 279, 1966.
(4) Heedman, P.A. and B. Jacobson. J. Clin. Endocrinol. 24: 246, 1964.
(5) Hickey, F.C. and G.L. Brownell. J. Clin. Endocrinol. 14: 1423, 1954.
(6) DeGroot, L.J. J. Clin. Endocrinol. 26: 149, 1966.
(7) Barzelatto, J., C. Beckers, C. Stevenson, E. Covatytubias, A. Gianetti, E. Bobadilla, A. Pardo, H. Dorosos, and A. Atria. Acta Endocrinol. 54: 577, 1967.
(8) Ermans, A.M., J.E. Dumont, and P.A. Bastenie. J. Clin. Endocrinol. 23: 539, 1963.
(9) Ermans, A.M., J.E. Dumont, and P.A. Bastenie. J. Clin. Endocrinol. 23: 550, 1963.
(10) Stanbury, J.B., G.L. Brownell, D.C. Riggs, H. Perinetti, J. Itoiz, and E.B. del Castillo. ENDEMIC GOITER. The Adaptation of Man to Iodine Deficiency. Cambridge, Harvard University Press, 1954.
(11) Weinstein, M., R.J. Soto, G. Sartorio, and A.H. Codevilla. J. Clin. Endocrinol. 27: 70, 1967.

factors), the iodination level of thyroglobulin and kinetic characteristics of the thyroid gland (intrinsic factors), all are important components of this regulating mechanism. The intrinsic factors are under enzymatic and hormonal control. The magnitude of the intrathyroidal iodine stores themselves seem to play an important role in determining the dynamics of iodine metabolism. There is experimental proof that the iodine content within the thyroid gland may effect the threshold level for the goitrogenic properties of TSH (1,2).

Our knowledge of total thyroidal iodine is based on destructive chemical studies in animals and surgical or autopsy specimen from humans. Biopsy specimen are too small to allow an adequate and representative sampling. Destructive techniques are still the reference method against which other tests of iodine quantitation will have to be compared.

Further advancement in our knowledge of total thyroidal iodine comes from studies of the kinetics of iodine metabolism based on a mathematical model using three interchanging pools and two forms of iodine (inorganic and organic). Details of this technique and the results have been reviewed extensively (3). In these studies equilibrium of a single bolus injection of radioactive iodine is reached between 10 and 14 days in normal subjects and in most of the goitrous patients. Then the total organic iodine pool can be calculated. Comparing the data obtained by chemical analysis (4) with those obtained by XRF analysis (reviewed and reported in this monograph) and those from the spectrophotometric method of Heedman et al. (5), it appears that in the normal thyroid gland and after more than 10 days of equilibration, the total exchangeable iodine pool and the total iodine content of the thyroid gland are equal. There are however exceptions.

Normal total iodine content varies widely in different subjects but is generally around 10 mg (Table 1). In two normal subjects on a standard diet and studied repeatedly over 210 days, the iodine content remained constant throughout this period (6)(Fig. 1).

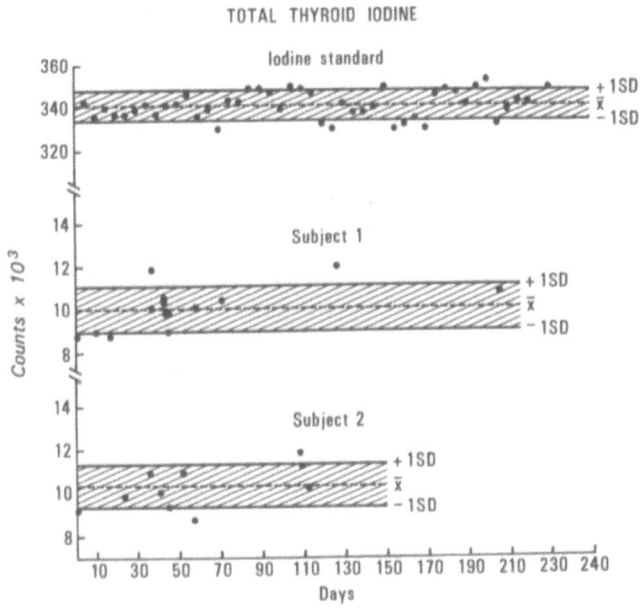

Figure 1. Longitudonal study of total iodine content is two normal subjects. Data from a simultaneously scanned phantom are given in the upper panel. (From reference 6 by permission).

The response of the iodine pool to oral iodine loading was evaluated by administering to a normal subject varying doses of potassium iodide and by monitoring the iodide pool with daily XRF measurements. Iodine content increased within 24 hours after a single dose of KI and gradually returned to previous levels. The increase in thyroid iodine was similar whether the single dose given was 1 mg or 100 mg, presumably

168

due to the uptake blocking effect of iodine. The return to
previous levels however was slower with the higher dose.
This could have been due to the longer time it takes to
clear the plasma from the extra iodine (Fig. 2).

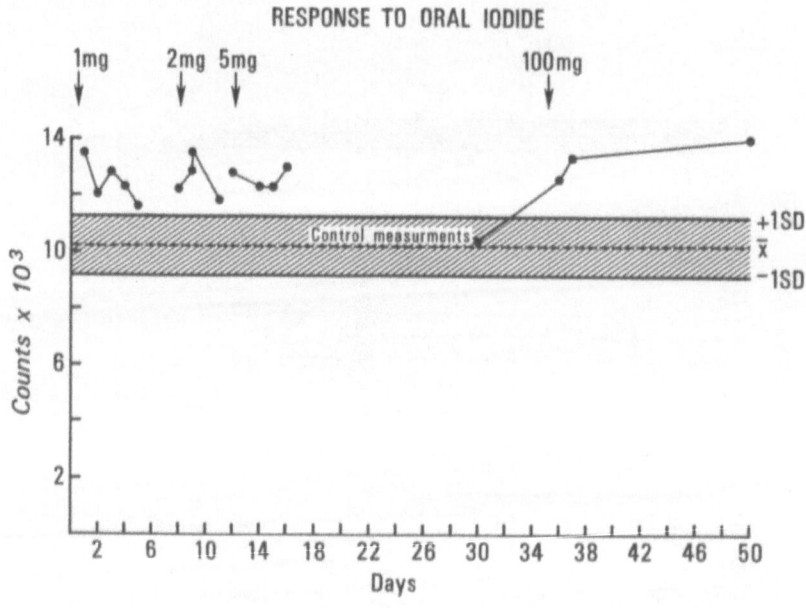

Figure 2. Total thyroid iodine in a normal subject taking
varying amounts of SSKI orally in a single dose.
Increase in thyroid iodine content shows little
relationship to the dose of oral iodine,
presumably because of the uptake blocking effect
of iodine. (From reference 6 by permission).

In a goitrous gland, iodine reserves vary in proportions
to the iodine supply. If there is no marked iodine
deficiency, as in sporadic goiter, the size of the
exchangeable iodine in the gland is often considerably
increased (5,7). In contrast, in endemic goiter, the total
exchangeable iodine pool remains about within the normal

range even if there is marked iodine deficiency (Table 1). Very low values of total exchangeable iodine have been reported in specific forms of endemic goiter (8,9), but chemical analysis suggested that in these cases the exchangeable iodine did not reflect the total iodine present. In large regions of Europe, urinary excretion of iodine is very low, reflecting insufficient dietary intake and very recently, at the 12th Meeting of the European Thyroid Association (E.T.A.), the low iodine urinary excretion in newborns was clearly demonstrated in the data (unpublished) presented by the Subcommittee of Neonatal Thyroid Screening of the E.T.A. In other regions of Europe, on the other hand, there is normal urinary excretion of iodine, however generally lower than in the U.S.A. While studying certain biochemical parameters of thyroid function in slices obtained from calves, discrepancies in iodine content were found between calf thyroids from Argentina and from North America, the latter showing a higher iodine content (10). These geographical differences in iodine content should be taken into account when discussing and comparing results of investigations concerning stable iodine metabolism.

When total iodine or iodine concentration are measured by XRF, low values are found in many cases of sporadic goiter (11, 4, 12, 13, 14). Proportionally more cases of sporadic goiter with low intrathyroidal iodine are found in areas where nutritional iodine supply is low, than in areas where iodine is adequately supplemented in the diet. This supports the impression that iodine deficiency is one of the causes of sporadic goiter (16). In locations where iodine is deficient or relatively deficient, XRF measurements may help to uncover the deficiency in those cases where a high uptake of radioiodine or radiotechnetium is found (small iodine pool, high turnover glands), as opposed to hyperthyroidism. This diagnosis is practically the only explanation for high suppressible thyroidal iodine uptakes in regions with known iodine deficiencies. Serum $T_4$, suppression test, TSH or TRH tests may be occasionally indicated to distinguish these glands from those with hyperthyroidism.

It has been shown that treatment with small doses of iodine can be beneficial in some cases of sporadic goiter (16) (see also Chapter VIII). An XRF measurement is essential to diagnose these cases. These cases may be spared the more classical treatment with thyroid hormones which further depletes the iodine stores (Figure 3)(11).

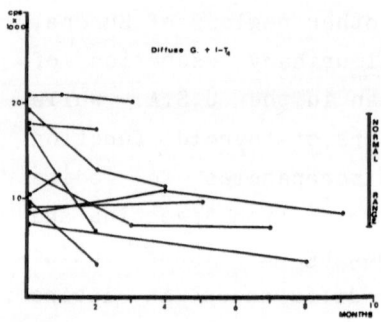

Figure 3.

Tendency of TITI to decrease in cases of sporadic goiter treated with $l-T_3$.

Total iodine content of the thyroid in different thyroid diseases has been studied by many investigators. An example of such a study is given in Figure 4. As a general rule the replacement of thyroid tissue by benign (Hashimoto's or lymphoid thyroiditis, acute thyroiditis) or malignant (differentiated and undifferentiated cancers) tissue leads to a reduction in the total iodine content and more pronounced to a reduction in regional iodine concentration. The fact that iodine content and concentration in the same thyroid disease varies in different patients has been shown repeatedly. This observation has generally been interpreted to suggest that XRF measurements do not significantly contribute to the diagnosis of thyroid disease. We are, however, of the opinion that this observation has not been sufficiently well exploited for its importance in understanding the mechanism of thyroid disease or for its value in diagnosis or management of disease. What for example is the difference between patients with high, normal or low iodine content who have Grave's Disease ? A few observations suggest that measurements of iodine content may indeed be interesting to pursue further.

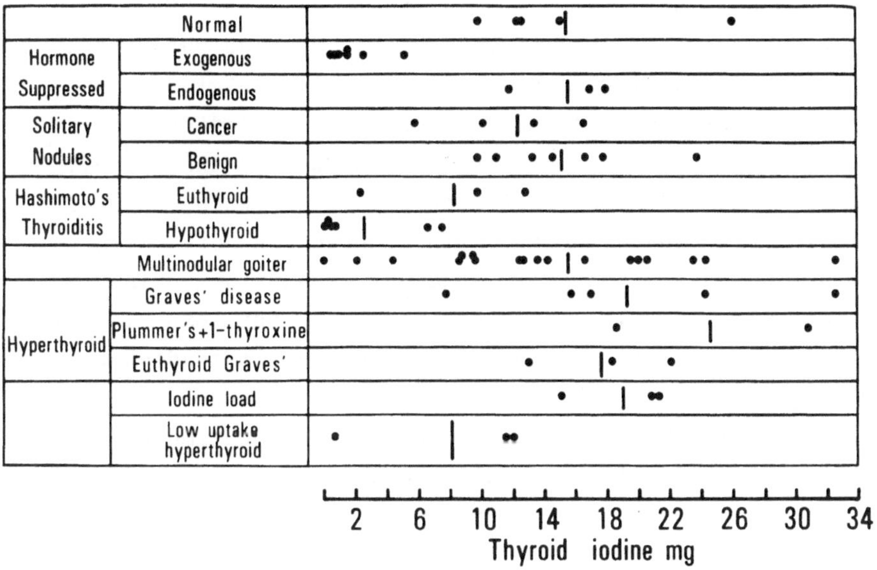

| | Normal | |
|---|---|---|
| Hormone Suppressed | Exogenous | |
| | Endogenous | |
| Solitary Nodules | Cancer | |
| | Benign | |
| Hashimoto's Thyroiditis | Euthyroid | |
| | Hypothyroid | |
| | Multinodular goiter | |
| Hyperthyroid | Graves' disease | |
| | Plummer's+1-thyroxine | |
| | Euthyroid Graves' | |
| | Iodine load | |
| | Low uptake hyperthyroid | |

Thyroid iodine mg (scale: 2 6 10 14 18 22 26 30 34)

Figure 4. Iodine content in 70 patients with thyroid disease and 5 normal subjects. (from reference 6 by permission).

Evidence has been published suggesting that the progressively decreasing intrathyroidal stores parallel and probably condition the incidious development of hypothyroidism in atrophic autoimmune thyroiditis (17, 18). XRF measurements have been helpful in our hands (11) when the results were found to be low, to stimulate more thorough investigations than would have been felt otherwise necessary to come to a definite diagnosis and also to decide whether or not substitution should be started.

Iodine contamination is more and more frequently encountered undoubtedly as a result of the extending availability and use of various radiological investigations involving iodinated contrast material. Iodine-containing drugs can also be the cause of high iodine intake, very often without the patient or the physician being aware of it. A survey made in 1979 showed that in only 30 out of the 139 iodine-containing drugs released in Belgium were sufficiently well labelled so that presence of iodine could be recognized from their name (iod-, iodo- and the like). Interviews demonstrated that most physicians were unaware of iodine in these drugs. The detection of iodine-contamination is classically done by measuring uriniary excretion of iodine. It is nevertheless our experience (M.J., unpublished data), that this approach is inadequate. After some radiological investigations, the urinary excretion of iodine may return to normal a long time before the iodine contamination can still be demonstrated by XRF of the thyroid. This fact can also be inferred from data presented in the literature (19).

In some instances, iodine contamination only induces anomalies of thyroid hormone metabolism at the periphery (20), without true dysthyroidism. In other instances iatrogenic hypo- or hyperthyroidism may result. Such examples are iodide goiter (21) or iodide-induced hyperthyroidism (see Chapter IX). These untoward reactions occur in already diseased glands (22). Hyperthyroidism has been shown to be a major complication of the massive administration of iodine in endemic areas in the months following the beginning of the treatment (23). These iatrogenic complications are less frequently found in regions where adequate dietary iodine has been available for a long time.

Before XRF became available, the presence of an enlarged iodine pool as the cause of disease in these particular cases could only be inferred from animal studies and by indirect means. Lately, direct proof of increased thyroid iodine stores was demonstrated in cases of iodide goiter (11). A relationship between increased iodine stores and **hyperthyroidism** (see Chapter IX) has been established. Subclinical hyperthyroidism as defined by pituitary unresponsiveness to TRH due to iodine overload has recently been documented (19, 24). These findings are of practical importance, but are only available to the physician if XRF facilities are available. In other cases the evolution of overt hyperthyroidism, closely linked to the iodine stores, treatment could be stopped the moment these stores reached normal levels (25). The differentiation between two forms of hyperthyroidism, one with high and another with low intrathyroidal stores, is probably of more practical importance in areas with low iodine intake. Persistance of high thyroidal iodine stores during treatment of hyperthyroidism has been shown to be of poor prognosis in the U.S. (15), an area of known high iodine intake.

Dysthyroidism due to amiodarone, a drug containing iodine amounting to 37% of its molecular weight (26), diserves a special comment because it illustrates the value of XRF measurements in some cases of iatrogenic thyroid disease. Table 2 shows the results of different parameters of thyroid function in 17 cases of patients treated chronically with amiodarone, observed lately in our department (M.J.). It can be seen that euthyroid remaining patients accumulate about 4 times as much iodine as normals, whereas some dysthyroid patients do not. It is felt that the inability of these glands to accumulate the drug, or the presence of low thyroidal iodine stores before treatment could be of prognostic significance (27). The same has been suggested for other drugs known to induce sporadic hypothyroidism (28).

Tabel 2. ITI and free hormones in amiodarone-taking patient.

1. Euthyroid
(n - 10)

| | m̄ ± s.d. | range |
|---|---|---|
| ITI (mg)<br>(N : 5.3 - 12.7) | 34.9 ± 23.6 | 21.0 - 100 |
| FT4 (ng/L)<br>(N : 6.60 - 14.0) | 15.36 ± 3.09 | 10.6 - 20.2 |
| FT3 (ng/L)<br>(N : 2.80 - 5.60) | 4.3 ± 1.25 | 3.0 - 7.6 |

2. Hyperthyroid

| | antibodies | ITI<br>(mg) | FT4<br>(ng/L) | FT3<br>(ng/L) |
|---|---|---|---|---|
| 1. | — | 28.0 | > 33 | 17.5 |
| 2. | — | 22.5 | 24.0 | 9.2 |
| 3. | — | 24.0 | 19.1 | 11.9 |
| 4 | + | 4.5 | 18.0 | 8.6 |

3. Hypothyroid

| | | | | |
|---|---|---|---|---|
| 1. | + | 1.5 | 3.4 | 2.0 |
| 2. | + | 15.0 | < 2.5 | 2.5 |
| 3. | + | < 1.5 | 4.8 | 2.1 |

# 3. LONGITUDINAL STUDIES OF TOTAL THYROIDAL IODINE

In normal subjects and in patients with thyroid disease
iodine uptake (measured by $^{131}$I, 24h uptake), synthesis of
thyroid hormone and hormone secretion are coupled. It is
therefore possible to estimate thyroid hormone secretion
from the uptake function i.e. high uptake of iodine usually
means elevated hormone secretion, in most cases.

In cases of lymphocytic thyroiditis with hyperthyroidism
however, uptake and hormone secretion functions are
uncoupled. Uptake function is blocked, but hormonal
secretion proceeds. In these cases radioactive iodine uptake
tests are not valid. Repeated measurements of total thyroid
iodine by XRF can however give an estimate of the rate of
decline of the iodine pool and this indirectly allows an

estimate of the hormonal secretion rate. The time a patient could be expected to remain hyper-thyroxinemic can also be estimated. These measurements are however not accurate enough to be useful for the calculation of the hormone secretion rate with an accuracy necessary for iodine turnover studies.

Because of the innocuousness of the method (ease of performance and low radiation burden), serial XRF measurements are ethically acceptable and were found to be useful in demonstrating the effect of treatment with low doses of iodine, even in children (Chapter VIII).

As stated above, XRF neasurements are useful in the follow-up of patients with hyperthyroidism that follows iodine contaminations, at least in some hands (11)(Chapter IX).

## 4. IODINE CONCENTRATION

There is a constant reduction in iodine concentration with increasing thyroid size in sporadic and endemic goiter (Table 1) and in all other thyroid diseases in which colloid filled follicular thyroid tissue is replaced by non-follicular tissue. In nodular goiters from endemic goiter region, stable iodine was lower in cold or functioning nodules than in paranodule tissue, but equal or higher in hyperfunctioning nodules (29). LeBlanc has evaluated thyroid cancer tissue and seen a similar result with respect to iodine content (4). These authors doubted therefore the usefulness of XRF in the approach to thyroid nodule. Patton et al. (30) have put this to the test and their results were not very promising. More convincing results are reported in Chapter IV, but the authors of the present section feel that the method is more one of statistical exclusion if iodine is found in a suspiscious lesion than of proof of malignity on the converse.

The advantages of expressing the results of XRF measurements in mgI/gr thyroid tissue instead of total iodine have been extensively discussed by Leisner during the symposium held in Brussels in September 1982 and alluded to in Chapter VIII of this monograph. It seems nevertheless that from the point of view of clinical applications, the choice is essentially a question of available facilities. Indeed, as a whole, comparable results in differential diagnosis and follow-up of patients have been obtained with both modes of expression. An unexpensive approach such as described in Chapter IV might be a practical solution.

## 5. RELATIONSHIP BETWEEN MORPHOLOGY AND IODINE CONTENT OR CONCENTRATION

In our study, measurable iodine by XRF was found only in thyroid tissue which contained follicles with colloid. There is however no strict relationship between the size of the follicle and the iodine content, since the iodination level of the thyroglobulin varies. The thyroid scan with XRF can therefore be considered a mapping of colloid bearing follicles regardless of their functional state.

This explains the discrepancy found between radioiodine scans and XRF mappings as shown in Chapter VII. It has already been remarked that such discrepancies are probably more frequent in western Europe than in the U.S. (10), underlyning once more that information from XRF assessments might be more relevant in areas with borderline alimentary iodine supplies. It certainly also underlines the fact that both methods do not yield the same information and therefore are not interchangeable.

Minor practical advantages of XRF can be commented upon. Because the method is dependant upon the presence of stable iodine, scans of the thyroid can be obtained in cases of iodine contamination and as it is independant of thyroid pituitary feedback, also when the patients are treated with thyroid hormones. Its low radiation burden allows morphological examination of the gland in pregnancy and during adolescence with less reluctance than would have been done with radioactive tracers. Scans have been obtained in patients who refused the administration of a radioactive product and in others who refused the intravenous route of these tracers.

## 6. SUMMARY AND CONCLUSIONS

The introduction of XRF technique for thyroid iodine quantitation and imaging allowed to verify results from previous kinetic studies and made it possible to evaluate iodine content in a number of diseases previously not investigated.

As judged from reports coming from areas where iodine is adequately supplemented in the diet, such as in the U.S.A., little usefulness was found as a whole for this method in everyday clinical practice within the framework of existing diagnostic categories. Future studies, however, are necessary before these measurements should altogether be dismissed. Reports from European countries, on the contrary, where urinary iodine is often low, probably due to unadequate iodine supply in the diet, differ in that respect. Besides that XRF allows a morphological evaluation of the thyroid gland in cases where the administration of radioactive tracers is unwarranted (pregnancy, adolescence), iodine content measurements were found especially useful in the diagnosis and follow-up of patients with thyroiditis (subacute and autoimmune atrophic) and hyperthyroid patients. XRF appear helpful to disclose iodine contamination and iatrogenic dysthyroidism due to iodine overload. If it could be confirmed that treatment of simple goiter with small doses of iodine is beneficial in some cases, XRF measurements could play a major role in the diagnosis and follow-up of these cases.

In conclusion, it is felt that XRF of the thyroid may be useful for the investigation of iodine metabolisms in thyroid disease in general, but that its place in the routine laboratory of a thyroid clinic will probably depend upon the geographical location and type of practice.

REFERENCES

01. Bray G.A. 1968. Increased sensitivity of the thyroid in iodine depleted rats to the goitrogenic effects of thyrotropin. J.Clin.Invest. 47: 1640.
02. Wahner H.W., Mayberry W.E., Gaitan E. and Gaitan J.E. 1971. Endemic Goiter in the Cancer Valley. III Role of Serum TSH in Goitrogenesis. J.Clin.Endocrinol.32: 491-496.
03. Stanbury J.B. (Ed.). 1968. Endemic Goiter, Report of a Meeting of the PAHO Scientific Group on Research in Endemic Goiter held in Puebla, Mexico in June 1968.
04. LeBlanc A.D., Bell R.L. and Jonhson P.C. 1973. Measurements of 127-I concentration in thyroid tissue by X-ray fluorescence. J.Nucl.Med. 14: 816-819.
05. Heedman P.A. and Jacobson B. 1964. Thyroid iodine determined by X-ray spectrophotometry. J.Clin.Endocrinol. 24: 246-252.
06. Wahner H.W., Sweet R.A., McConahey W.M. and Duick D.S. 1978. Fluorescent thyroid scanning. A method based on stable iodine measurements. Mayo Clin.Proc. 53: 151-156.
07. Ermans A.M. 1969. Intrathyroidal Iodine Metabolism in Goiter. In: Endemic Goiter, Report of a Meeting of the PAHO Scientific Group on Research in Endemic Goiter held in Puebla, Mexico. Stanbury J.B. (Ed.): 1-13.
08. Ermans A.M., Dumont J.E., Bastenie P.A. 1963. Thyroid function in an endemic goiter. I. Impairment of hormones synthesis and secretion in the groitrous gland. II. Non-hormonal iodine escape from the goitrous gland. J.Clin.Endocrinol. & Metab. 23: 539-560.
09. Stanbury J.B., Brownell G.L., Riggs D.C., Pennettic H. Itoiz J. and del Castillo E.B. 1954. Endemic Goiter. The adaptation of men to iodine deficiency. Cambridge, Harvard University Press.
10. Pisarev M.A., Kleiman de Pisarev D.L. 1980. Biochemistry of thyroid regulation under normal; and abnormal conditions. J.Endocrinol.Invest. 3: 317-329.
11. Jonckheer M.H. and Deconinck F. 1982. X-ray fluorescence determination of stable iodine in the thyroid gland. A review. Acta Clinica Belgica 37: 92-102.

12. Leisner B., Kantlehner R., Heinze.. et al. 1979.
    Klinische Ergebnisse der Schilddrusenszintigraphie und
    Jodbestimmung mit Fluorezenstechnik. Forsch. Geb.
    Roentgenstr. Nuklearmed. 130: 694-699.
13. Rappaport B., Block M.B., Hoffer P.B. et al. 1973.
    Depletion of thyroid iodine during subacute thyroiditis.
    J.Clin.Endocrinol. & Metab. 36: 610-611.
14. Thrall J.H., Gillen M.T., Johnson M.C. et al. 1978.
    Quantificative thyroid fluorescent scanning technique
    and clinical experience. Am.J.Rontgenol. 130: 517-522.
15. Hoffer P.B., Bernstein J., Gottschalk A. 1971.
    Fluorescent techniques in thyroid imaging.
    Semin.Nucl.Med. 1: 379-389.
16. Ermans A.M., Verelst J. 1980. Acute effects of supra-
    physiological doses of iodine in the human being:
    management of non-toxic goiter. J.Mol.Med. 4: 199-202.
17. Jonckheer M.H., Vanhaelst L., Deconinck F., Michotte Y.
    1981. Atrophric Autoimmune Thyroiditis: Relationship
    between the Clinical State and Intrathyroidal Iodine as
    Measured in Vivo in Man. J.Clin.Endocrinol. & Metab. 53:
    476-479.
18. Jonckheer M., Coomans D., Massart D.L., Vanhaelst L.,
    Deconinck F. 1982. The application of SIMCA pattern
    recognition to the study of autoimmune atrophic
    thyroiditis. Nucl.Med.Com. 3: 70-77.
19. Habermann J., Leisner B., Witte A., Pickardt C.R.,
    Scriba P.C. 1982. Iodine contamination as a cause of
    hyperthyroidism or lack of TSH response to TRH
    (Results based on a screening investigation).
    J.Endocrinol.Invest. 5: 153-156.
20. Burger A.G., Lambert M., Cullen M. 1981. Interference de
    substances medicamenteuses dans la conversion de T4 en
    T3 et rT3 chez l'homme. Annales Endocrinol. 42: 461-469.
21. Wolff J. 1969. Iodide goiter and the pharmacologic
    effects of excess iodide. Am.J.Med. 47: 101-124.
22. Braverman L.E., Woeber K.A., Ingbar S.H. 1969. Induction
    of myxoedema by iodine in patients euthyroid after
    radioiodine or surgical treatment of diffuse toxic
    goiter. New Eng.J.Med. 281: 816-821.
23. Adams D.D., Kennedy T.H., Stewart J.C., Utiger R.D.,
    Vidor G.I. 1975. Hyperthyroidism in Tasmania Following
    Iodide Supplementation: Measurements of Thyroid-
    Stimulating Autoantibodies and Thyrotropin.
    J.Clin.Endocrinol. & Metab. 41: 221-228.
24. Musch W., Jonckheer M.H., Segers O., Coomans D.,
    Goldstein J., Van Steirteghem A.C., Vanhaelst L. 1982.
    Increased stable intrathyroidal iodine pool as a cause
    of pituitary unresponsiveness to TRH stimulation. Ann.
    Endocrinol. (Paris) 43: 49A (Abstract).
25. Jonckheer M.H., Deconinck F., Swaenepeol L. 1980. Upon
    the importance of differentiating between two forms of
    hyperthyroidism by means of X-ray fluorescence scanning.
    In: Stockligt Jr., Nagataki S. (Eds). Thyroid Research
    VIII. Australian Academy of Sciences, Canberra,
    Australia: 637-640.

26. Broeckhuyzen J., Larnel R., Sion R. 1969. Recherches dans la serie des benzofurances XXXVII. Etude comparee du transit et du metabolisme de l'amiodarone chez diverses especes animales et chez l'homme. Archives Intern. de Pharmacodyn. 177: 340.
27. Jonckheer M.H. 1981. Amiodarone and the thyroid gland. A review. Acta Cardiol. 36: 199-205.
28. Jonckheer M.H. 1980. Iatrogenic hypothyroidism. In: Bastenie P.A., Bonnijns M., Vanhaelst L. (Eds). Recent progress in diagnosis and treatment of hypothyroid conditions. Excerpta Medica, Congress Series (Amsterdam) 529: 15-28.
29. Wahner H.W., Gaitan E., Correa P. 1966. Studies on Iodine Metabolism in Endemic Nodular Goiter. J.Clin.Endocrinol. 26: 279-286.
30. Patton J.A., Hollifield J.W., Brill A.B., Lee G.S., Patton D.D. 1976. Differentiation between malignant and benign solitary thyroid nodules by fluorescent scanning. J.Nucl.Med. 17: 17-21.

Author Index                                    Pages

# SUBJECT INDEX